Diagnostic Ultrasound in the Dog and Cat

KV-140-129

LIBRARY OF VETERINARY PRACTICE

EDITOR

S. T. SWIFT
MA, VetMB, CertSAC

LIBRARY OF VETERINARY PRACTICE

Diagnostic Ultrasound in the Dog and Cat

FRANCES BARR MA, VetMB, DVR, MRCVS
Department of Veterinary Surgery
University of Bristol
Langford House, Langford
Bristol BS18 7DU

Blackwell
Science

© 1990 by
Blackwell Science Ltd
Editorial Offices:
Osney Mead, Oxford OX2 0EL
25 John Street, London WC1N 2BL
23 Ainslie Place, Edinburgh EH3 6AJ
350 Main Street, Malden
  MA 02148 5018, USA
54 University Street, Carlton
  Victoria 3053, Australia
10, rue Casimir Delavigne
  75006 Paris, France

Other Editorial Offices:

Blackwell Wissenschafts-Verlag GmbH
Kurfürstendamm 57
10707 Berlin, Germany

Blackwell Science KK
MG Kodenmacho Building
7–10 Kodenmacho Nihombashi
Chuo-ku, Tokyo 104, Japan

The right of the Author to be identified as the Author
of this Work has been asserted in accordance with
the Copyright, Designs and Patents Act 1988.

All rights reserved. No part of
this publication may be reproduced,
stored in a retrieval system, or
transmitted, in any form or by any
means, electronic, mechanical,
photocopying, recording or otherwise,
except as permitted by the UK
Copyright, Designs and Patents Act
1988, without the prior permission
of the publisher.

First published 1990
Reprinted 1992, 1995, 1998

Set by Setrite Typesetters, Hong Kong
Printed and bound in Great Britain by
The University Press, Cambridge

The Blackwell Science logo is a
trade mark of Blackwell Science Ltd,
registered at the United Kingdom
Trade Marks Registry

DISTRIBUTORS

Marston Book Services Ltd
PO Box 269
Abingdon
Oxon OX14 4YN
(*Orders*: Tel: 01235 465500
          Fax: 01235 465555)

USA
Blackwell Science, Inc.
Commerce Place
350 Main Street
Malden, MA 02148 5018
(*Orders*: Tel: 800 759 6102
                781 388 8250
          Fax: 781 388 8255)

Canada
Login Brothers Book Company
324 Saulteaux Crescent
Winnipeg, Manitoba R3J 3T2
(*Orders*: Tel: 204 224 4068)

Australia
Blackwell Science Pty Ltd
54 University Street
Carlton, Victoria 3053
(*Orders*: Tel: 03 9347 0300
          Fax: 03 9347 5001)

British Library
Cataloguing in Publication Data

Barr, Frances
  Diagnostic ultrasound in the dog
  and cat.
  1. Pets. Dogs. Diagnosis.
  Ultrasonography   2. Pets. Cats
  Diagnosis. Ultrasonography
  I. Title   II. Series
  636.7089607543

ISBN 0-632-02845-9

Contents

Preface

Diagnostic ultrasound is an imaging technique which has much to offer in veterinary medicine. However, in order to gain as much information as possible from an ultrasonographic examination, it is essential firstly to obtain good quality images, and secondly to be familiar with the normal appearance of the various body tissues. Only then may the departures from normality associated with disease or injury be appreciated.

The aim of this book is to provide a practical guide to the ultrasonographic examination of the dog and cat. The photographs have been chosen to demonstrate normal and abnormal structures, while the accompanying line drawings are designed to clarify images which may be confusing to the inexperienced eye. As with any essentially practical technique, there can be no substitute for personal experience, but this book is designed to provide a basis on which to begin using diagnostic ultrasound. As the veterinary surgeon becomes more experienced in the use of this technique, I hope that the text and illustrations will remain useful as a source of reference.

FRANCES BARR
Department of Veterinary Surgery
University of Bristol

Publisher's note

Whilst the advice and information contained in this book are believed to be true and accurate at the date of going to press, neither the author nor the publisher can accept any legal responsibility or liability for any errors or omissions that may be made.

Acknowledgements

I would like to acknowledge the cooperation of my colleagues in the Departments of Veterinary Surgery and Medicine in encouraging the ultrasonographic examination of clinical cases under their care. Particular thanks are due to Dr. C. Gibbs and Dr. P. Wotton, who performed some of the examinations illustrated in this book. My colleagues in the Department of Pathology have been very helpful in establishing the final diagnosis in many of the cases.

I would also like to thank Professor H. Pearson, Dr. S. Crispin, Dr. P. Wotton and Mr. A. Barr for their constructive comments during the preparation of the text. Mr. A. Barr took the photographs illustrated in Figs 2.2, 3.1, 3.15, 6.1 and 8.1. Many thanks are due to Mr. Conibear for preparing the photographic illustrations.

Figures 1.7, 3.6 and 6.11 are reproduced by kind permission of the publishers of *In Practice*. Figures 3.6 and 4.3 were originally published in *The Veterinary Annual*, volume 28 (1988) and are reproduced by permission of the publishers, Butterworth and Co. (Publishers) Ltd, who retain copyright in this material. Figure 3.7 is reproduced by kind permission of the publishers of *Veterinary Radiology*.

I am grateful for the financial support provided by the Alison Alston Canine Award (awarded by the Royal College of Veterinary Surgeons) and the BSAVA Clinical Studies Trust Fund for the last three years, allowing me to study ultrasound as a diagnostic technique.

Finally, thanks to my husband Alistair for his continuous encouragement and support.

FRANCES BARR

1/Principles of Diagnostic Ultrasound

Production of the image

Diagnostic ultrasound is an imaging technique which makes use of high-frequency sound waves. Frequencies currently employed range from 2 to 10 MHz, whereas the highest frequency audible to the normal human ear is only about 20 kHz.

The ultrasound transducer contains one or more crystals with piezo-electric properties. If a voltage is applied across the crystal, it undergoes mechanical deformation and consequently emits sound waves of a characteristic frequency. This is termed the inverse piezo-electric effect (Fig. 1.1). Within the transducer, a voltage is applied intermittently across the crystal so that short pulses of high-frequency sound, lasting only a few microseconds, are emitted.

If the transducer is placed in contact with the body surface, the sound waves pass into the tissues. Different tissues have a different resistance to the passage of sound, or acoustic impedance. The average velocity of sound waves through soft tissues is about 1540 m/s, through bone around 4000 m/s, and

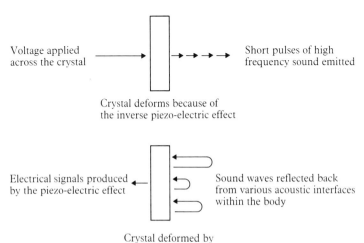

Voltage applied across the crystal   Short pulses of high frequency sound emitted

Crystal deforms because of the inverse piezo-electric effect

Electrical signals produced by the piezo-electric effect   Sound waves reflected back from various acoustic interfaces within the body

Crystal deformed by returning echoes

Fig. 1.1 How the transducer works.

through air approximately 300 m/s. Whenever the sound waves meet an interface between two tissues of differing acoustic impedance, part of the sound is reflected. Where the difference in impedance is great (e.g. soft tissue−air or soft tissue−bone) a large part of the sound is reflected and little goes on into deeper tissues. Where the difference in impedance is small (e.g. soft tissue−soft tissue) only a small proportion is reflected and most of the sound continues into deeper tissues. If the interface is perpendicular to the incident sound beam, the reflected echo will travel directly back to its source. Interfaces at an angle to the incident sound waves produce scattered reflections. Thus, the strength of a returning echo depends on the difference in impedance at the interface and also the angle of that interface relative to the sound beam. As the sound beam travels through the tissues it gradually becomes weaker (attenuated), owing to a combination of reflection, scatter and absorption.

The reflected sound is detected by the same crystal. This is possible since the interval between the pulses of emitted ultrasound is sufficiently long to allow the echoes from one pulse to return and be analysed before the next pulse is sent out. The returning echoes cause mechanical deformation of the crystal and thus the production of electrical signals by the piezo-electric effect. These signals are analysed according to the strength and depth of reflection, and displayed on a screen.

Image display modes

A mode (amplitude mode)

This is the simplest form of image display. A single fixed beam of ultrasound is used, and the returning echoes are shown as peaks along a horizontal line. The height of each peak denotes the strength of the echo, while the horizontal axis represents the depth of the reflecting structure (Fig. 1.2). This display mode is little used now as it provides only limited information about organ boundaries.

B mode (brightness mode)

Multiple beams of ultrasound are used, and the echoes from each beam are analysed. The returning echoes are represented as a dot on the screen, the position on the screen representing

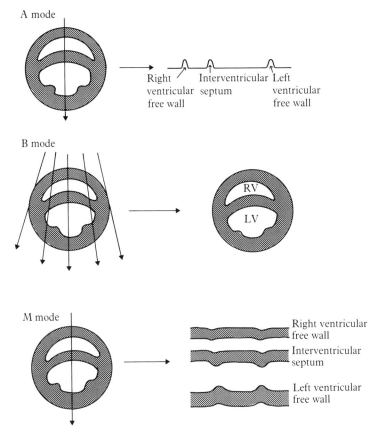

A mode

Right ventricular free wall   Interventricular septum   Left ventricular free wall

B mode

RV

LV

M mode

Right ventricular free wall

Interventricular septum

Left ventricular free wall

Fig. 1.2 Diagrammatic illustration of A, B and M mode images of the heart. RV = right ventricle, LV = left ventricle.

the position of the reflecting structure within the body. The strength of the echo is shown by the brightness of the dot on the screen. Thus, a two-dimensional image representing a slice through the body is built up and displayed on the screen (Fig. 1.2). In the early days of B mode imaging, only strong echoes could be represented. This meant that the edges of structures were shown but little internal architecture. In the 1970s technological advances allowed the display of a wider range of image brightness, enabling both small echoes arising from within an organ, and strong echoes from organ boundaries, to be displayed. This is termed grey-scale imaging.

The original compound B scans (static scans, articulated arm scans) used a transducer mounted on an articulated arm. The image was built up by moving the transducer sequentially over the body surface. This allowed a large field of view, but was a fairly time-consuming procedure requiring some patient cooperation. The image achieved was static. Moving structures could clearly not be imaged using this technique.

Static B scans have now largely been superseded by real-time scanning. In real-time scanning, many sound beams are emitted sequentially by either an array of crystals or a single moving crystal. The cross-sectional image is assembled and displayed very rapidly, and is then updated continuously, allowing movement of structures within the section to be seen. Real-time is now the most commonly used ultrasound display mode in both human and veterinary medicine.

M mode (motion mode)

A single ultrasound beam is used, and the returning echoes are displayed as a series of dots along a vertical line. The position of the dot along that line represents the depth of the reflecting structure, and the brightness of the dot denotes the strength of the echo. This line is continuously updated as the screen scrolls horizontally. The resulting image represents movement of structures along the line (Fig. 1.2). The particular value of M mode displays lies in cardiology. Some transducers are dedicated to M mode and emit only a single ultrasound beam. Perhaps of more use in veterinary medicine are the real-time transducers which produce a cross-sectional image, but which allow selection of a single scan line and M mode display when required.

Transducer characteristics

The crystal

The thickness of the crystal determines the frequency of sound it generates. The diameter of the crystal varies according to the purpose for which the transducer is intended. The wider the diameter of the crystal for a given frequency, the more it can be focussed. This allows finer lateral resolution, but the transducer itself will be larger and consequently more cumbersome.

The sound beam

The transducer crystal produces sound of a characteristic frequency. The higher the frequency of sound produced, the finer is the resolution achieved, but the greater is the attenuation in the body tissues. Therefore, a high-frequency transducer should be selected to image structures where resolution of fine detail is of paramount importance but deep penetration of tissues is not needed (e.g. 7.5–10 MHz for examination of the eye). A low frequency transducer is chosen when fine resolution is of less importance than deep tissue penetration (e.g. 3.5–5 MHz for examination of thoracic and abdominal viscera in large dogs).

Early clinical use of ultrasound showed that focussing of the ultrasound beam was of great importance as the unfocussed sound beam diverges rapidly and poor resolution is achieved. The focal zone of a transducer is that part of the sound beam where focussing, and consequently image resolution, is optimal (Fig. 1.3). In the near field of the sound beam, or *Fresnel zone*, complex diffraction patterns may occur. Beyond the focal zone the beam begins to diverge rapidly and resolution diminishes. This is termed the *Fraunhofer zone*. The clinical relevance of this is that it is important to place the structure under examination within the focal zone, by appropriate selection of the transducer and adaptation of the scanning technique if necessary. A stand-off may be used to increase the distance between the transducer and the skin surface and thus bring the organ of interest into the focal zone. A stand-off may be composed of any material which is echolucent and does not attenuate the sound beam, e.g. a water-filled bag or a block of semisolid gel. It may be a separate feature or an integral part of the transducer.

Annular array transducers are now becoming popular. In these transducers the crystal is divided into concentric rings of varying thickness. Different frequencies of sound are produced and the sound beam can be focussed over a greater depth than is possible with other systems.

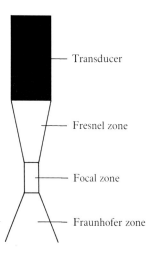

Fig. 1.3 The focussing of the sound beam.

Transducer type

Two main types of ultrasound transducer are widely available (Fig. 1.4):

Linear array transducer

These transducers usually have between 60 and 256 crystals arranged in a line. Small groups of crystals are operated in turn, giving a rectangular field of view. Electronic focussing can be used to improve image resolution. The main advantage of these types of transducer is that they allow a large field of view, even close to the scanning surface, which facilitates

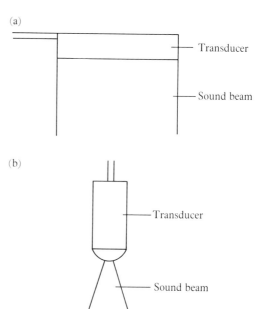

Fig. 1.4(a) A linear array transducer produces a rectangular sound beam. (b) A sector transducer produces a fan-shaped sound beam.

recognition of structures and the anatomical relationship between them. The major disadvantage is that they require a relatively large contact area with the body surface. This is particularly true of those transducers initially designed for use in human obstetrics, which are so bulky as to be virtually useless in small animals. The most recent linear array transducers designed for veterinary use are much smaller and this problem is thus minimized.

Some linear array transducers are designed with a convex scanning surface. This gives a mildly diverging field of view, but the advantages and disadvantages of these curved linear array transducers are much the same as for the flat design.

Sector transducer

These transducers produce a fan-shaped field of view. A wide-angled fan allows more structures to be seen but gives poorer resolution than a smaller-angled fan:

1 Mechanical sector scanners have a small number of crystals which are driven mechanically to sweep out a fan-shaped beam. This is achieved by mounting a small number of crystals on a rotating wheel, or by using a single crystal which oscillates to and fro.

2 Phased array sectors use a fixed array of crystals which are electronically triggered to sweep the ultrasound beam through a fan-shaped field.

The sector scanners in general have the advantage of being small and easy to use, and they require only a small skin contact area. However they have a smaller field of view, making it more difficult to identify and relate structures. The near field is particularly restricted. Nevertheless, sector transducers are generally preferable to linear array transducers for use in small animals because of their size and manoeuvrability. The phased array sector transducers are undoubtedly technically superior to the mechanically driven sector transducers — the resolution is better, there are no moving parts to wear out, and they do not produce a sense of vibration when applied to the skin. However they are currently more expensive.

Equipment controls

The number and complexity of controls on diagnostic ultrasound machines vary enormously. Common facilities are listed below, but few machines will have all these controls:

1 On−off switch.

2 Transducer selection (linear array vs. sector; frequency).

3 Display mode selection (B mode vs. M mode).

4 Power output. The power control is usually calibrated in decibels, and regulates the amount of sound emitted by the transducer, and thence the strength of the returning echoes. This alters the overall brightness of the image. Too little power results in loss of fine detail while too much power obliterates detail, because of too many echoes. As a general guide, the lowest power which still allows good differentiation of structures should be used.

5 Time Gain Compensation (TGC). (Also termed *Depth Gain Compensation* (DGC) or swept gain controls.) Ideally, identical targets should produce echoes of the same strength irrespective of their position within the body. However, the sound beam becomes attenuated as it passes through the tissues, so deeper structures will produce weaker echoes than superficial structures. The gain controls allow electronic amplification of the returning echoes to compensate for this reduction in signal strength with depth. The actual controls vary from machine to machine, but the aim is to adjust the gain until there is an even image density throughout the field (Fig. 1.5). There is

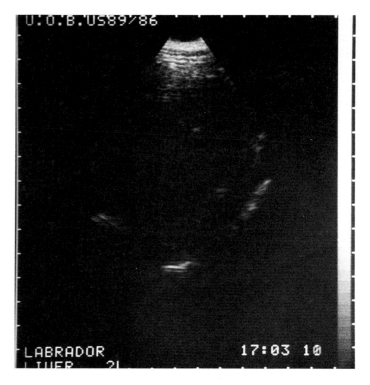

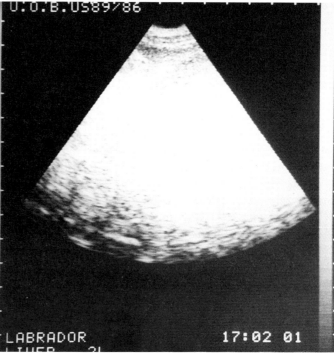

Fig. 1.5 Incorrect use of gain controls. (a) shows the image with the overall gain set too low. The diaphragm line can just be seen, but no details of the liver parenchyma are visible. (b) shows the image with the overall gain set too high. The resulting 'noise' obliterates virtually all details of the image.

usually a graphical representation of the gain curve on the screen.

6 *Pre- and post-processing controls.* These controls can be used to alter the image by accentuating different levels of echoes and so enhancing organ boundaries or fine architectural details. The preprocessing controls act before the image is displayed, while the postprocessing controls are used to modify the frozen image on the screen. Such controls should be used with great care as it is possible to produce artefacts and eliminate true lesions.

7 Freeze frame (for freezing the image on the screen).

8 Electronic callipers (allowing measurement of the distance between two points and the circumference and area of an object).

9 Magnification or zoom (allowing magnification of part of the image).

10 *Beam angle.* There may be the option of altering the angle of the sector imaged. With wider angles there is a larger field of view, but either a slower scanning speed or inferior resolution.

11 *Frame rate.* It may be possible to select the frame rate, allowing a slower rate for improved resolution, or a faster rate to allow full appreciation of moving structures.

12 *Split frame.* Some machines allow the display of two images side by side — either two cross-sectional images or one cross-sectional image and one M mode image.

13 ECG — allowing simultaneous display of the ECG trace and ultrasound image.

Image recording

All modern ultrasound equipment allows the displayed image to be frozen. It is of great importance that there is the facility to record this frozen image, as this allows subsequent examination and discussion of the image and enables accurate comparisons to be made on follow-up examinations. It also allows a library of the ultrasonographic appearance of normal and diseased organs to be compiled. There are a number of options available for recording the frozen image:

1 *Polaroid camera.* This is a simple and initially cheap system, whereby the camera is swung in front of the screen to photograph the frozen image. The major disadvantage is that the polaroid images are of poor quality. In addition, each print is expensive to produce.

2 *Video printers*. These imagers have fairly recently become available. They are initially more expensive to buy than a polaroid camera, but produce rapid reproductions of the frozen image on paper at very little cost. The prints are of excellent quality, although they unfortunately have the tendency to turn yellow-brown with time.

3 *Multiformat camera*. These cameras may be automatic or manual, but both types are expensive to purchase. Images are produced on X-ray film, which is processed routinely to produce a permanent image of excellent quality. The cost of producing each image is low, as four to six images may be recorded on each piece of film. The multiformat camera is certainly the method of choice for recording the frozen image, but the initial cost may sometimes place it out of reach.

It is also very useful to be able to record the moving image. The simplest way to do this is to link a video recorder to the screen, which allows recording of the scanning procedure and subsequent replay. This is probably essential for a full cardiac evaluation but is also useful for other ultrasonographic examinations.

Patient preparation

It is rarely necessary to anaesthetise small animals for ultrasonographic examination. However, it is helpful if the animal is reasonably cooperative, and it may be necessary to sedate very nervous or aggressive animals. In cardiac evaluation it may be better to avoid sedation as the heart rate and motility may be affected.

Depending on the organ under examination, an appropriate 'acoustic window' should be selected. In other words, an area of the body surface should be chosen overlying the organ of interest and avoiding intervening bone and structures containing gas. Bone or gas will at best impair image quality, and at worst block the sound beam completely.

Meticulous preparation of the scanning area is essential. Good contact between the transducer and skin must be achieved for optimal image quality (Fig. 1.6). In most cases this entails careful clipping of the coat from the scanning area, although occasionally the coat of a long-haired breed of dog or cat can simply be parted. The skin should then be carefully cleaned with surgical spirit to remove dirt and excessive grease. Finally, liberal quantities of a commercial acoustic gel should be applied to ensure good contact between

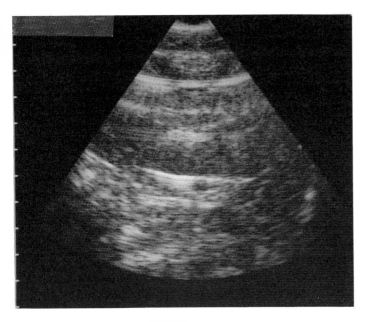

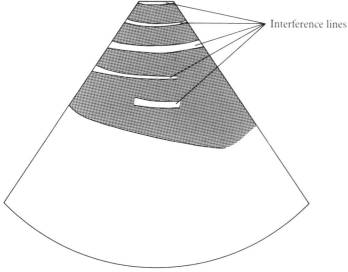

Interference lines

Fig. 1.6 The white lines running horizontally across the image are indicative of poor skin-transducer contact. As a result, the image quality is very poor.

the skin and the transducer. Alternatives to commercial gels, such as liquid paraffin or cooking oil, have been used with some success, but it is important to check that the use of these alternatives does not invalidate service maintenance contracts or purchase guarantees.

Having prepared the scanning area, the transducer may then be placed in contact with the skin and the investigation started.

Principles of image interpretation

In the early days of medical ultrasound, images were some-times displayed as white on a black background and sometimes as black on a white background. Thus both formats may be found in the literature. It is now conventional to use a white image on a black background.

A number of terms may be used to describe the image:

Hyperechoic; echogenic:	Bright echoes, appearing white on conventional scans. Represent highly-reflective interfaces, e.g. bone, gas, collagen.
Hypoechoic; echopoor:	Sparse echoes, appearing dark grey on conventional scans. Represent intermediate reflection/transmission, e.g. many soft tissues.
Anechoic; echolucent; sonolucent; transonic:	Absence of echoes, appearing black on conventional scans. Represent complete transmission of sound, e.g. fluid.

Bone and gas prevent the passage of sound. At a soft tissue−gas interface, around 99% of the sound is reflected. At a soft tissue−bone interface, around 30% of the sound is reflected but the remainder of the sound is strongly absorbed. Thus in both cases a strong echo is produced from the surface but structures beneath the surface are not imaged.

Fluid is generally anechoic although the presence of particulate matter within it may produce echoes. Soft tissues appear as various shades of grey depending on their cellular composition and the type and number of internal interfaces. Collagen is known to be a potent source of internal echoes. Fat has a more variable ultrasonographic appearance but is most often echogenic. As well as assessing the overall echo-genicity of tissues, the echo texture can be evaluated (the size, density and distribution of internal echoes).

Common imaging artefacts

It is important to be able to recognize the common imaging artefacts so that misinterpretation may be avoided.

Acoustic shadowing

As already discussed, bone and gas block the passage of sound. This results in an intensely echogenic line at the surface of such structures, but nothing beneath the surface is seen. This is the phenomenon of acoustic shadowing (Fig. 1.7). Recognition of this effect may be useful in the detection of small calculi in the kidney, bladder or gall bladder.

Acoustic shadowing may also occasionally be recognized distal to the margins of a rounded fluid-filled structure (e.g. gall bladder), resulting from refraction of the sound beam.

Acoustic enhancement

Sound waves pass unimpeded through fluid, so there is often a particularly bright area immediately beneath the fluid. This is the phenomenon of acoustic enhancement (Fig. 1.8). Recognition of this effect may be useful in confirming the fluid nature of an area on the image.

Reverberation

Reverberation artefacts occur at highly reflective interfaces. The strong echo returns to the transducer, where it is reflected and re-enters the body tissues. This may occur several times, resulting in multiple images parallel to and beneath the original interface (Fig. 1.9). This type of artefact is most often seen at soft tissue or fluid interfaces with gas. It is not often seen at soft tissue—bone interfaces because the bone absorbs the sound efficiently.

One particular type of reverberation artefact is the comet-tail artefact, so called because of the stream of reverberations trailing beyond the original interface.

Mirror-image artefact

This artefact also occurs at highly reflective interfaces. In this instance, multiple internal reverberations occur between the interface and other body tissues. Thus some echoes are delayed in returning to the transducer and are displayed as originating beyond the original interface (Fig. 1.10). There are two instances in veterinary ultrasonography when the mirror-image artefact is common. The diaphragm—lung interface is highly reflective and a mirror image of the liver may be seen beyond

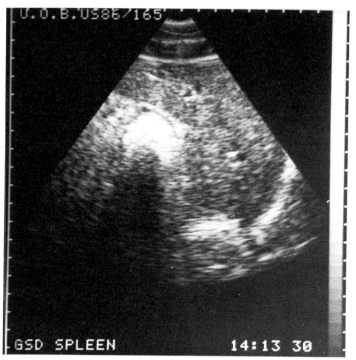

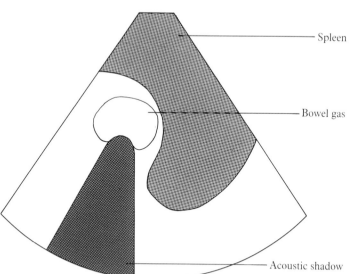

Fig. 1.7 An accumulation of gas within the bowel produces an intensely echogenic area which casts a clear acoustic shadow.

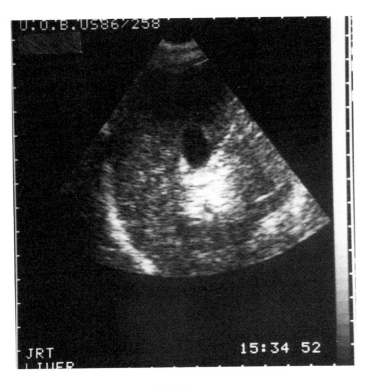

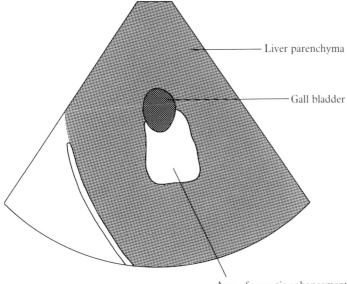

Liver parenchyma

Gall bladder

Area of acoustic enhancement

Fig. 1.8 A bright area of acoustic enhancement is visible deep to the gall bladder.

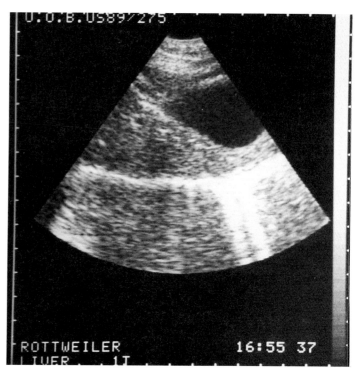

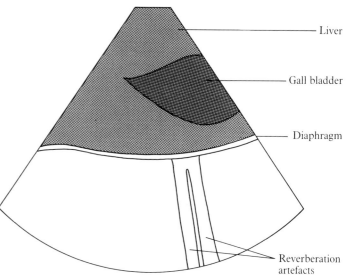

Fig. 1.9 Two bright streams of reverberations are seen, originating at the highly reflective interface between the lung and the diaphragm.

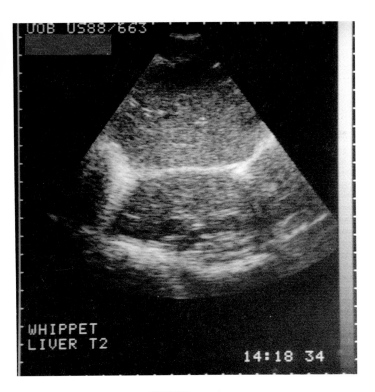

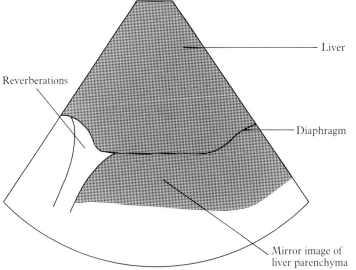

Fig. 1.10 A mirror image of the liver parenchyma can clearly be seen beyond the diaphragm.

the diaphragm. It is important to recognise this as an artefact rather than a pathological disruption of the integrity of the diaphragm. The pericardium–lung interface is also highly reflective, and a mirror image of the heart is sometimes seen.

Doppler ultrasonography

Simple Doppler ultrasound has been used for some years in veterinary medicine as a means of pregnancy diagnosis. Tremendous advances have recently been made in the field of Doppler imaging, which expand the potential applications of this technique enormously. The images which may be produced and the artefacts which commonly arise will not be covered in this volume, but a short discussion of the principles involved will clarify the potential uses of Doppler ultrasonography.

Doppler ultrasonography allows the measurement of the velocity of blood flow in vessels or chambers of the heart. Once the velocity distribution of blood flow has been determined, the type of flow (laminar or turbulent) may be defined and pressure gradients estimated.

High-frequency sound waves are emitted and pass into the tissues of the body. When the reflecting interface is moving with respect to the transducer, there is a change in the wavelength and a corresponding change in the frequency of the reflected sound. This frequency change is termed the Doppler shift. The frequency shift is determined by the frequency of emitted sound, the velocity of the reflecting surface and the velocity of sound in the tissues. The Doppler shift encountered in clinical situations usually lies in the frequency range of 100 Hz – 11 kHz, representing a velocity range of 10 – 100 cm/s.

When the motion of the reflector is not parallel to the sound beam, then only the vector component in that direction is considered. This gives a frequency shift which corresponds to a velocity less than the actual velocity, simply due to the angle. Therefore the angle of incidence of the sound beam must also be considered in any calculations.

Continuous wave Doppler

The transducer crystal emits a continuous beam of ultrasound. A separate transducer receives the echoes, and compares the frequency with that transmitted. The frequency shift may be displayed graphically and/or audibly. These systems allow measurement of a wide range of velocities, but provide no positional information as a moving object anywhere along the beam may produce the signal.

Pulsed wave Doppler

Ultrasound is emitted by the transducer in pulses and the returning echo is received by the same transducer. Because the delay is related to the depth of the reflecting structure, it is possible to determine the position of the source of the Doppler shift. However, the pulsatile transmission limits the maximum velocity which may be measured.

Duplex Doppler imaging

This technique combines pulsed Doppler with two-dimensional real-time imaging, allowing precise localization of the Doppler sample. Most systems use two transducers within a single probe for duplex imaging. The cross-sectional image and the graphical Doppler display are shown simultaneously on the screen.

Colour flow Doppler

This system allows velocity information for the whole cross-sectional image to be displayed. This information is added to the two-dimensional image as colour, with the colour and intensity depicting the direction and magnitude of the velocity. Such a technique clearly offers enormous potential as it provides functional as well as anatomical information, but the equipment is currently very expensive.

The biological safety of diagnostic ultrasound

The effects of diagnostic ultrasound on living tissues have been intensively investigated. Ultrasound has been widely used in human medicine, particularly in the field of obstetrics, for more than 10 years, and there have been no substantiated reports of adverse clinical effects. Early reports of chromosomal damage to human leucocytes after diagnostic exposure were not confirmed. It is known that high-intensity ultrasound can damage DNA *in vitro* and impair cell growth. However, diagnostic ultrasound employs the pulse echo principle so that total exposure of body tissues is low. In the light of present knowledge, it seems that diagnostic ultrasound is biologically safe and without adverse clinical effects.

Further reading

Barr, F. (1988) Diagnostic ultrasound in small animals. *In Practice*, **10**, 17–25.

Herring, D.S. and Bjornton, G. (1985) Physics, facts and artefacts of diagnostic ultrasound. *Veterinary Clinics of North America: Small Animal Practice*, **15**, 1107–1126.

Nelson, T.R. and Pretorius, D.H. (1988) The Doppler signal: where does it come from and what does it do? *American Journal of Roentgenology*, **151**, 439–447.

2/Imaging of the Liver and Spleen

The liver

Imaging procedure

In the dog and cat the liver normally lies within the costal arch with the stomach immediately behind it. It is important therefore that the stomach should be empty when the liver is to be examined as even moderate quantities of food and/or gas will interfere with the passage of sound and prevent a thorough inspection of the liver (Fig. 2.1). Barium sulphate in the stomach will also adversely affect image quality. However, a stomach filled with fluid does not impair image quality, and may indeed act as a useful landmark.

The animal is placed in dorsal recumbency. A padded foam trough or a blanket will make the animal more comfortable and therefore less inclined to struggle. An area of hair is clipped from the ventral abdomen between the xiphisternum and the umbilicus, extending several centimetres on each side of the midline. After routine preparation of the site, the transducer is placed just behind the xiphisternum and angled cranially and dorsally until the liver is identified (Fig. 2.2). Sweeps of the transducer are then made from right to left and from dorsal to ventral until the entire substance of the liver has been examined. If the liver is enlarged the transducer may need to be moved back towards the umbilicus to ensure that the whole liver is seen.

There are a number of other possible approaches to examination of the liver in small animals and it may be necessary to try several methods until optimal images are produced. If stomach or bowel gas interferes with image quality when the animal is in dorsal recumbency, better images may be produced with the animal in lateral recumbency or standing. Gas tends to rise and it is possible to take advantage of this by intelligent positioning of the animal so that gas is displaced from the organ of interest.

In very deep-chested dogs, or if the liver is very small, it

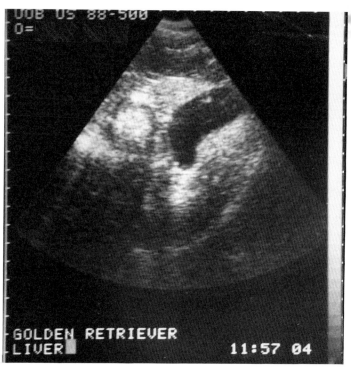

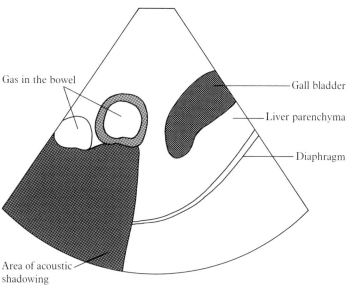

Fig. 2.1 Gas within the gastrointestinal tract causes acoustic shadowing, thus preventing a complete evaluation of the liver.

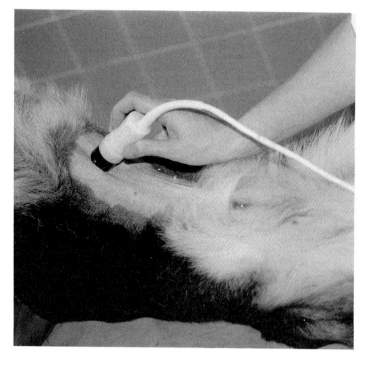

Fig. 2.2   Imaging of the liver.

may be difficult to see the liver with the transducer behind the xiphisternum. In such cases an intercostal approach is useful. The animal is placed in lateral recumbency with the right side uppermost. (If the left side is uppermost gas tends to rise into the gastric fundus, preventing adequate visualization of the liver.) An area of hair is clipped over the ventral third of the last three or four ribs. After the skin has been prepared the transducer is placed in each intercostal space in turn until the best view of the liver is obtained. Although this technique allows a reasonable view of the liver, it is not possible to make such a systematic examination of the whole parenchyma as with the previously described methods.

Normal appearance

The normal liver has a similar ultrasonographic appearance in the dog and cat (Fig. 2.3). The diaphragm is clearly visible as a thin, distinct, echogenic line which moves up and down with respiration. It thus acts as a useful and easily recognizable landmark. The liver lies between the diaphragm and the skin surface.

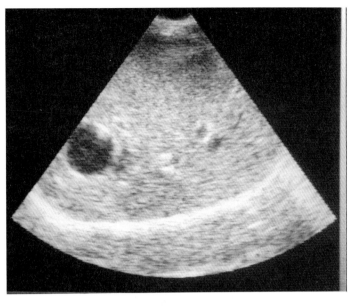

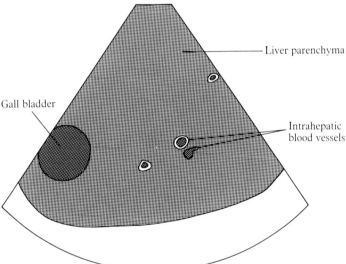

Gall bladder

Liver parenchyma

Intrahepatic
blood vessels

Fig. 2.3 Normal liver in a Greyhound. The gall bladder is clearly seen.

The ultrasonographic appearance of the liver parenchyma is coarsely granular, but with a uniform texture throughout. With correct adjustment of the gain controls, the liver is usually moderately hypoechoic. In order to assess hepatic echogenicity objectively it is necessary to compare the liver with other parenchymal organs at the same depth and control settings (Figs 2.4 and 2.5).

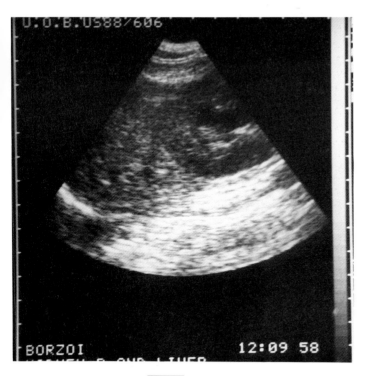

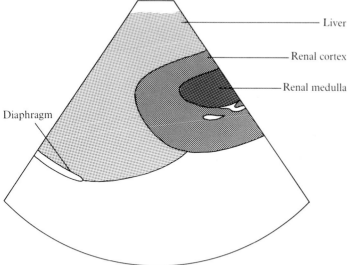

Liver

Renal cortex

Renal medulla

Diaphragm

Fig. 2.4 Normal liver and kidney in a Borzoi. The renal cortex is usually slightly less echogenic than the liver.

Renal cortical echogenicity ≤ hepatic echogenicity ≤ splenic echogenicity. Localized patches of echogenicity in an otherwise orderly liver are quite frequently seen and probably represent areas of fibrous tissue (falciform ligament, interlobar fissures etc.).

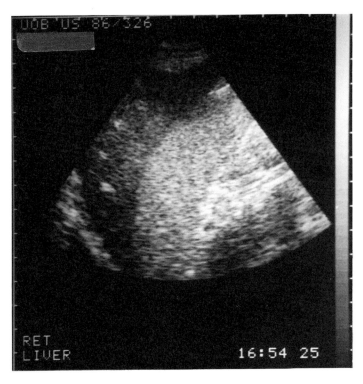

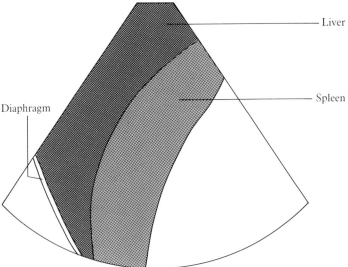

Fig. 2.5 Normal liver and spleen in a Golden Retriever. The spleen is usually more echogenic and more densely textured than the liver.

The gall bladder is usually seen to the right of the midline within the hepatic parenchyma. It is a smooth, clearly-defined, round or oval structure with thin walls and anechoic contents. The phenomenon of acoustic enhancement can be recognized deep to the gall bladder. The size of the gall bladder is very variable depending on when the animal has last eaten. With current limits of resolution the intrahepatic bile ducts are not usually seen.

Intrahepatic blood vessels can be identified as anechoic channels seen in both longitudinal and cross sections (Fig. 2.6). Portal veins have strongly echogenic margins, because of

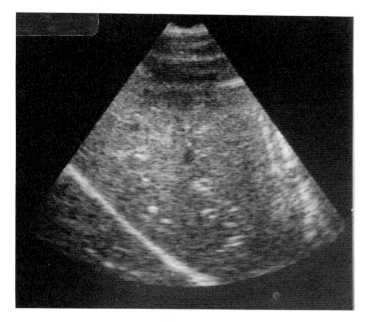

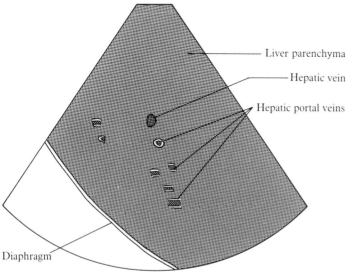

Liver parenchyma

Hepatic vein

Hepatic portal veins

Diaphragm

Fig. 2.6 Normal liver in a Springer Spaniel. The normal liver parenchyma is evenly hypoechoic. Intrahepatic vessels can be identified — hepatic portal veins have echogenic walls, and most hepatic veins do not have echogenic walls.

the fibrous tissue of the portal tracts, while hepatic veins in general do not have echogenic walls. The largest hepatic veins may have echogenic walls, but these vessels can usually be followed to their junction with the caudal vena cava. The caudal vena cava is a large vessel identified at the hilus of the liver, and it can be followed as it passes through the diaphragm at this point. Hepatic arteries cannot normally be identified with current instrumentation.

Focal parenchymal lesions

Focal parenchymal disease is recognized by localized disruption of the normally uniform texture of the liver (Figs 2.7 and 2.8). Such disruptions should be carefully examined and the following features noted:

1 Number — single or multiple?
2 Shape.
3 Size.
4 Boundary definition.
5 Echogenicity — increased, decreased or mixed?

Neoplasia, whether primary or secondary, is probably the commonest cause of focal hepatic parenchymal lesions in man and small animals. Focal patterns commonly associated with hepatic neoplasia in man include:

1 Discrete relatively echolucent masses.
2 Discrete relatively echogenic masses.
3 Bull's-eye lesion (dense centre, lucent periphery).
4 Mixed.

All of these patterns have been recognized in the dog but types 1 and 4 are most commonly seen. Depending on their echogenicity, lesions smaller than 1–2 cm in diameter are not reliably identified. Lesions of homogeneous cellularity and low vascularity (e.g. lymphosarcoma) tend to have low echogenicity. Necrosis and liquefaction in the centre of large tumour masses also gives rise to hypoechoic areas. Hypervascular masses and areas of fibrosis, calcification or haemorrhage tend to give rise to hyperechoic lesions. However, it is not possible to predict the histological nature of a lesion from the ultrasonographic appearance — biopsy is required for a definitive diagnosis.

Focal hepatic lesions are not, however, necessarily neoplastic. Benign nodular hyperplasia in man may give rise to areas of either increased or decreased echogenicity. Few reports mention the ultrasonographic appearance of this condition in small

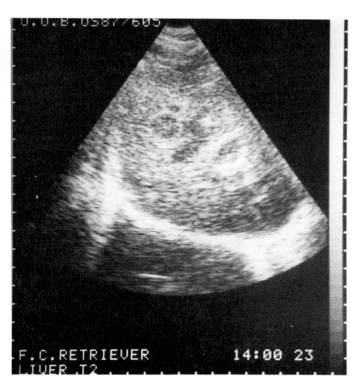

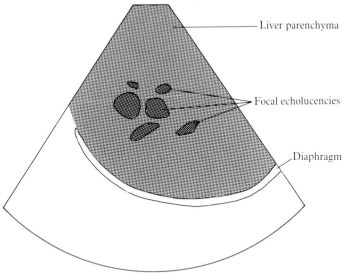

Liver parenchyma

Focal echolucencies

Diaphragm

Fig. 2.7 Hepatic lymphosarcoma in a Flat Coat Retriever. Multiple, focal, hypoechoic areas are seen scattered through the liver parenchyma. These represent small lymphosarcomatous nodules.

animals, but it seems likely to be just as non-specific as in man.

Fresh intraparenchymal haemorrhage, which is usually a result of trauma, gives rise to echogenic foci. Subsequently

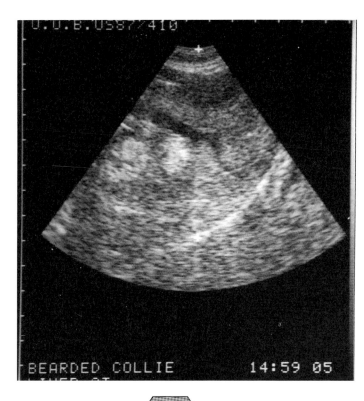

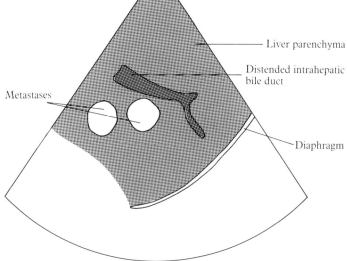

Liver parenchyma

Distended intrahepatic bile duct

Metastases

Diaphragm

Fig. 2.8 Extrahepatic biliary obstruction due to a pancreatic carcinoma, with hepatic metastases, in a Bearded Collie. Focal, rounded echogenicities within the liver parenchyma represent the metastatic lesions. The irregular, branching, fluid-filled tube is a distended intrahepatic bile duct.

the ultrasonographic appearance of haematomata varies as they age. As the clot forms and retracts the lesion may become predominantly anechoic. As organization progresses a mixed echogenicity is seen. Sequential examination should show a progressive decrease in size as the haematoma resolves.

Intrahepatic abscesses usually have thick, irregular, ill-defined walls. The contents vary from hypoechoic to moderately echoic depending on the thickness of the pus and the presence of debris. This appearance is not specific however and may also be seen with necrotic tumours or haematomata.

Hepatic necrosis or infarction results in areas of decreased echogenicity. If subsequent resolution results in scar formation then such areas will be of increased echogenicity.

Hepatic cysts are not common in small animals, but should have a characteristic appearance of a sharply defined, rounded, anechoic mass with marked posterior acoustic enhancement.

In summary, focal parenchymal lesions in the liver of small animals are often readily identified. The ultrasonographic changes seen however are rarely specific and so tissue biopsy or aspiration is necessary to allow a definitive diagnosis to be made.

Diffuse parenchymal disease

Diffuse hepatic disease may be much more difficult to identify sonographically. There may be a generalized disturbance of the normal even echo texture, with a mixture of echogenicities giving a patchy or mosaic appearance (Fig. 2.9). Such findings may be associated with both diffuse neoplasia and with advanced cirrhosis, so biopsy will be required for a definitive diagnosis.

It is important to examine the edges of the liver, which should be very smooth. An irregular or nodular margin is certainly not normal but is a non-specific finding. It is easier to detect such abnormalities in the presence of abdominal fluid as this separates and outlines the lobes (Fig. 2.10).

More often in diffuse hepatic disease there is no detectable disturbance of architecture. The ultrasonographic appearance may be normal, or there may be subtle changes in overall echogenicity. Such changes can only be appreciated by critical comparison of the relative echogenicities of the liver, spleen and renal cortex at the same depth and control settings. In man an increase in hepatic echogenicity has been associated with both cirrhosis and other chronic liver disease, and with fatty infiltration. A relative decrease in parenchymal echogenicity with accentuated periportal echogenicity has been linked with acute hepatitis and cholecystitis. It is likely that

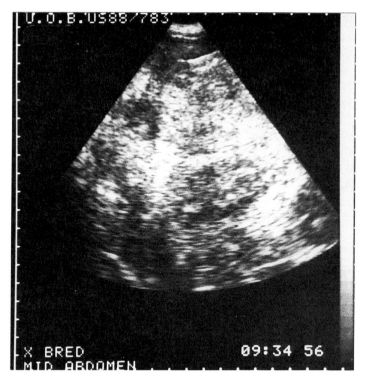

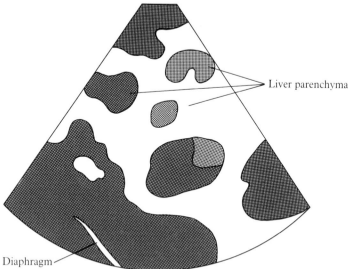

Fig. 2.9 Diffuse hepatic neoplasia in a cross-breed dog The liver parenchyma is extremely heterogeneous in density and texture.

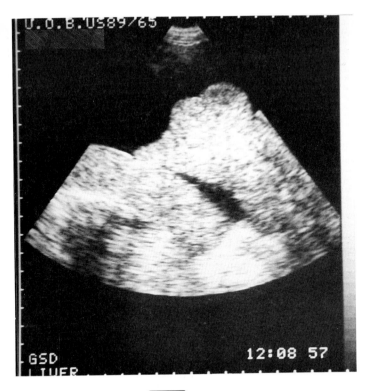

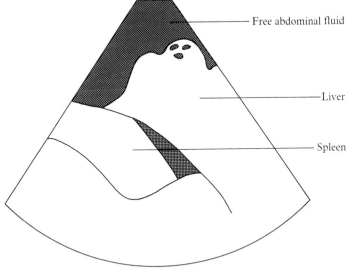

Free abdominal fluid

Liver

Spleen

Fig. 2.10 Hepatic haemangiosarcoma in a German Shepherd Dog. The free fluid, which in this case is blood, separates and outlines the liver lobes. Thus, the irregular, nodular margin of one liver lobe is clearly seen.

similar changes may occur in small animals, but no comprehensive studies have been reported to date. A homogeneous decrease in echogenicity has been described in some cases of hepatic lymphosarcoma in the dog. It must be emphasized that these changes in echogenicity are non-specific, so biopsy is needed for a definitive diagnosis.

The gall bladder and biliary system

The normal gall bladder has a thin smooth wall and anechoic contents. When there is bile stasis secondary to fasting or anorexia, or in cases of acute hepatic dysfunction with reduced bile outflow, the bile may become more echogenic and consequently difficult to distinguish from the surrounding parenchyma (Fig. 2.11).

Cholecystic calculi are not common in small animals but are easily detected ultrasonographically. They are echogenic particles which tend to fall to the dependent portion of the gall bladder, casting strong acoustic shadows.

The gall bladder wall may become thickened producing a double ring. In man this has been attributed to acute or chronic cholecystitis (where the thickening is inflammatory), but is also seen associated with severe hypoalbuminaemia and heart failure (where the thickening is largely due to oedema). Similar changes have been reported in the dog ascribed to cholecystitis and to hypoalbuminaemia.

Perhaps the most common indication for ultrasonographic examination of the biliary system in small animals is to differentiate extrahepatic obstructive jaundice from other types of jaundice. Experimentally it has been shown that total acute biliary obstruction in the dog leads to dilation of the gall bladder and common bile duct (24–72 h) followed by enlargement of the intrahepatic bile ducts (from about 6 days onwards). Partial obstructions are likely to produce a longer time course. Dilated intrahepatic bile ducts can be differentiated from portal vessels by their rather tortuous paths and less regular branching patterns (see Fig. 2.8). In the absence of discernible dilation of the biliary tree, jaundice is more likely to be of hepatocellular or prehepatic origin.

The vascular system

Intrahepatic venous abnormalities are often readily recognized on ultrasonographic examination. The commonest abnormality

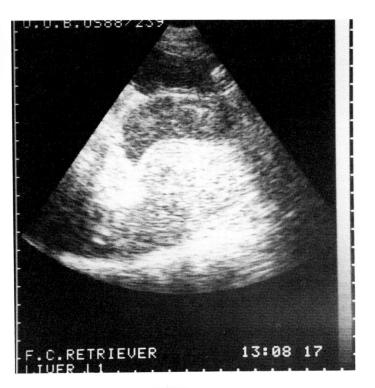

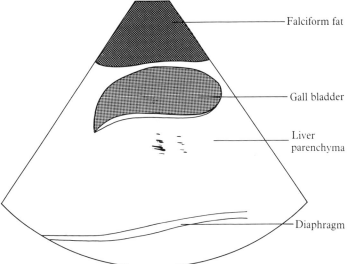

Fig. 2.11 Acute hepatic dysfunction in a Flat Coat Retriever. The bile within the gall bladder contains echoes, reflecting bile stasis. The gall bladder wall is also thicker than normal.

seen in small animals is hepatic venous congestion, resulting from right-sided cardiac failure. Similar congestion may occur secondary to obstruction of the caudal vena cava between the liver and the heart. Although hepatic veins are visible in the normal liver, they appear more numerous and more distended in hepatic venous congestion (Fig. 2.12). At present this remains a subjective evaluation as the normal range in size of hepatic veins in small animals has not been established. Ascites in the absence of hepatic venous distension is likely to be of non-cardiac origin.

Portosystemic shunts in small animals can sometimes be identified ultrasonographically. Examination of these animals can be difficult however as the liver tends to be very small and consequently obscured by the gastrointestinal tract. It has been suggested that ultrasonography of such cases should be performed under general anaesthesia with intermittent positive pressure ventilation. This tends to displace the liver caudally, but also leads to an increase in central venous pressure and distension of the caudal vena cava and intrahepatic veins, facilitating recognition of abnormal shunting vessels. The type of shunt which is most readily identified is a patent ductus venosus. An abnormal large tortuous or sigmoid vessel is seen in the liver near the hilus running into the caudal vena cava — although its precise path is often difficult to follow (Fig. 2.13). Primary extrahepatic shunts cannot usually be identified. In acquired liver disease secondary venous shunting may occur, and in such cases large tortuous blood vessels may be recognized in the abdomen caudal to the liver.

The ultrasonographic findings associated with congenital hepatic arteriovenous fistulas in dogs have been described. Anechoic irregular lakes or tortuous tubular structures in or adjacent to liver parenchyma were seen.

Detailed consideration of colour flow Doppler techniques are beyond the scope of this text. However, such techniques allow assessment of the direction and velocity of blood flow, and when available in conjunction with real-time scanning, allow a more accurate evaluation of the hepatic vascular system.

The spleen

Imaging procedure

The spleen is a very mobile organ, and may be found in a number of orientations in the abdomen. The head of the spleen however, is relatively fixed adjacent to the greater curvature of the stomach in the left cranial abdomen. Consequently, it is often easier to locate the head of the spleen initially.

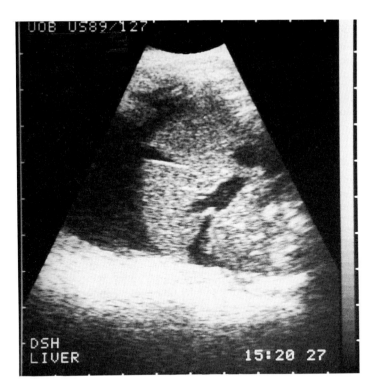

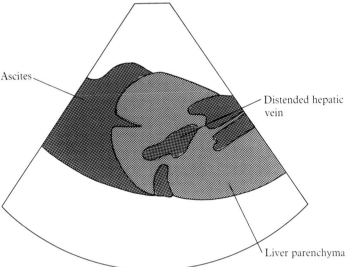

Fig. 2.12 Hepatic venous congestion in a cat. Large amounts of free abdominal fluid are visible, separating the liver lobes. Distended hepatic veins within the liver parenchyma can also be seen.

The animal is placed in dorsal recumbency. A large area of hair must be clipped from the ventral abdomen, from the xiphisternum to midway between umbilicus and pubis. The area should extend several centimetres to each side of the

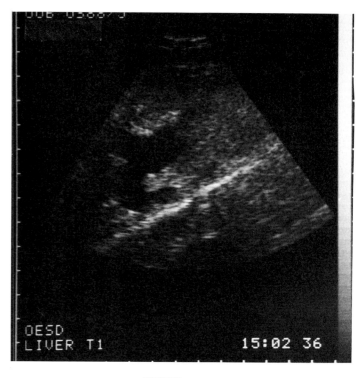

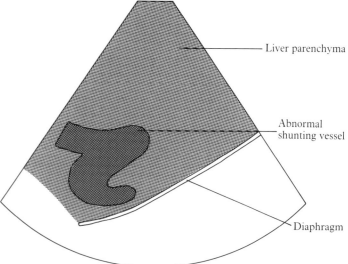

— Liver parenchyma

Abnormal shunting vessel

Diaphragm

Fig. 2.13 Patent ductus venosus in an Old English Sheepdog. A large, sigmoid, shunting vessel is visible within the substance of the liver.

midline. After routine skin preparation the transducer is placed just behind the xiphisternum, perpendicular to the skin. The transducer is then slowly moved along the costal arch to the left until the head of the spleen is located. The stomach should preferably be empty or fluid-filled so that the gastric contents do not interfere with image quality. In some animals the transducer may need to be angled slightly cranially under the costal arch to see the spleen. Conversely, gastric distension or hepatomegaly may result in caudal displacement of the head of the spleen. Having identified the head of the spleen, it is then possible to follow the body and tail either' along the left flank or running obliquely across the abdominal floor. It is very important to examine the spleen meticulously throughout its length, in order to minimize the risk of missing abnormalities.

The spleen may also be examined with the animal in right lateral recumbency, but it may then be more difficult to follow the organ throughout its length.

The spleen generally lies very close to the abdominal wall, and this must be borne in mind during the imaging procedure. Undue application of pressure during scanning may result in the spleen slipping sideways away from the transducer head. A more important consideration is that optimal imaging may not be achieved unless the transducer is designed to focus within the first 3−4 cm. A stand-off may be useful to bring the spleen within the focal zone of the transducer.

Normal appearance

The spleen in the dog is normally smooth and well-defined in outline. The head is roughly triangular in cross-section, while the body and tail become progressively flatter in shape. In the cat the normal spleen is a very slender strap-like organ and may not always be identified.

The size of the spleen varies greatly in normal animals, even within one individual, owing to its function as a circulatory reserve. It is well known, for example, that marked splenomegaly may occur during barbiturate anaesthesia. Thus, assessment of splenic size seems at present to be of little clinical value in small animals.

Ultrasonographically, the splenic parenchyma has a densely granular appearance, of even texture throughout (Fig. 2.14). When compared with the liver, the spleen is usually slightly more echogenic, and the granularity is finer and denser. This echogenicity can be ascribed to the highly vascular nature of the organ. However, individual vessels are not usually identified except at the hilus.

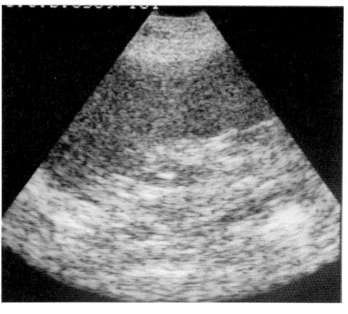

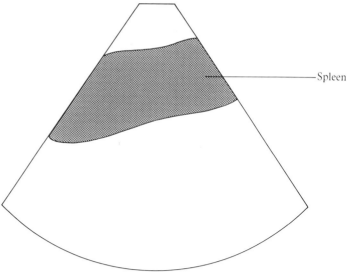

—Spleen

Fig. 2.14 Normal spleen in a
Basset Hound.

Focal parenchymal lesions

Focal disturbances of the normal even echo texture of the
spleen are readily recognized if a meticulous examination of
the organ is made (Figs 2.15 and 2.16). The size, shape and
echogenicity of any abnormalities should be noted, as well as
the clarity of the boundary between normal and abnormal

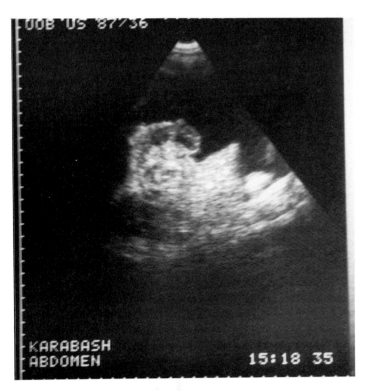

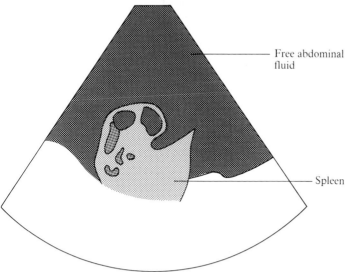

Free abdominal fluid

Spleen

Fig. 2.15 Splenic haemangiosarcoma in an Anatolian Karabash. The free abdominal fluid, which in this case is blood, delineates a fungating mass of mixed echogenicity protruding from the surface of the spleen.

areas. It is also important to decide whether lesions are single or multiple.

Probably the most common focal abnormalities seen in the spleen in small animals are neoplasms. Depending on their

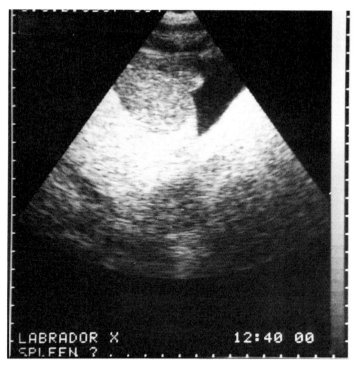

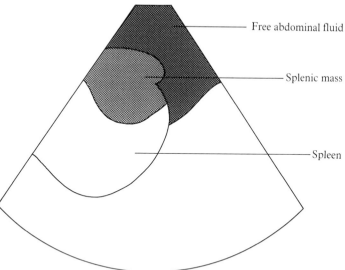

Free abdominal fluid

Splenic mass

Spleen

Fig. 2.16 Splenic haemangiosarcoma in a cross-breed dog. The free fluid outlines the spleen. A well-circumscribed mass of moderate, even echogenicity is visible within the splenic parenchyma and protruding from one margin.

echogenicity, lesions as small as 1 cm may be detected. Splenic tumours vary greatly in their ultrasonographic appearance, but in small animals they are usually either evenly hypoechoic or of mixed echogenicity. It is not generally possible to predict accurately the histological type of tumour from the ultra-sonographic appearance.

Trauma of the spleen may occasionally result in complete transection of the organ. More often, lacerations and contusions result in intraparenchymal and/or subcapsular haemorrhage. These haematomata are usually of mixed echogenicity, but vary in appearance according to the stage of clot formation, retraction and resorption. Sequential ultrasonographic examinations should show gradual resorption of simple haematomata. However, splenic haemangiomata and haemangiosarcomata have a particular tendency to bleed, and may also result in large intraparenchymal and subcapsular haematomata. Associated free abdominal fluid is also frequently present. Thus it may be impossible to differentiate a simple splenic haematoma from a bleeding splenic haemangioma or haemangiosarcoma ultrasonographically unless metastases are detected in other organs.

Splenic abscesses are not common in dogs and cats. Classically they have thick irregular walls and contents which vary in echogenicity. The presence of gas which is due to gas-forming organisms renders the contents highly echogenic, and acoustic shadows may be cast. However, an abscess cannot usually be distinguished ultrasonographically from either a tumour with a necrotic centre or an organizing haematoma.

Infarcts of the spleen may occasionally be recognized. In the early stages these are hypoechoic or of mixed echogenicity. With scar formation, infarcts become typically hyperechoic and wedge-shaped.

Thus focal lesions of the spleen can usually be identified but the ultrasonographic appearance is rarely specific. The history and clinical examination may suggest a likely interpretation, and ultrasonographic examinations of other organs may provide additional information. Fine needle aspiration of lesions may be helpful in some cases to clarify the diagnosis, but is said to be contraindicated where haemangiosarcoma is suspected because of seeding of malignant cells along the needle tract.

Diffuse parenchymal disease

Focal splenic neoplasms may become so large that they replace all the normal parenchyma. In such cases it is difficult to determine with certainty the organ of origin of the mass — the absence of a normal spleen and the identification of other

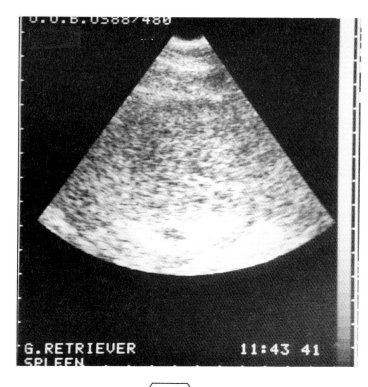

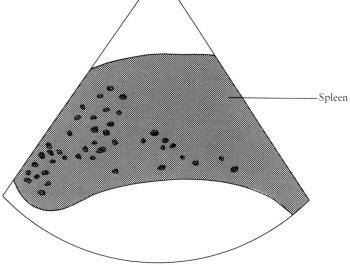

Spleen

Fig. 2.17 Diffuse splenic lymphosarcoma in a Golden Retriever. The normal homogeneous, dense texture of the spleen has been replaced by a slightly 'moth-eaten' appearance, resulting from many tiny hypoechoic patches.

abdominal organs allow a presumptive diagnosis of a splenic mass.

Diffuse infiltrative neoplasms of the spleen generally cause no discernible ultrasonographic abnormality other than a smooth enlargement of the entire organ. The echotexture is usually undisturbed. In some cases the overall echogenicity of the spleen when compared with the liver and kidney cortex may be altered (Fig. 2.17).

Generalized splenomegaly may occur in association with septicaemia or toxaemia. Smooth enlargement of the spleen may also be seen with passive venous congestion secondary to right-sided heart failure, general anaesthesia or chronic liver disease, or in cases of vascular compromise (eg. splenic torsion).

Further reading

Bailey, M.Q., Willard, M.D., McLoughlin, M.A., Gaber, C. and Hauptman J. (1988) Ultrasonographic findings associated with congenital hepatic arteriovenous fistula in three dogs. *Journal of the American Veterinary Medical Association*, **192**, 1099–1101.

Cartee, R.E. (1981) Diagnostic real time ultrasonography of the liver of the dog and cat. *Journal of the American Animal Hospitals Association*, **17**, 731–737.

Feeney, D.A., Johnston, G.R. and Hardy, R.M. (1984) Two dimensional gray-scale ultrasonography for assessment of hepatic and splenic neoplasia in the dog and cat. *Journal of the American Veterinary Medical Association*, **184**, 68–81.

Nyland, T.G. (1984) Ultrasonic patterns of canine hepatic lymphosarcoma. *Veterinary Radiology*, **25**, 167–172

Nyland, T.G. and Gillett, N.A. (1982) Sonographic evaluation of experimental bile duct ligation in the dog. *Veterinary Radiology*, **23**, 252–260.

Nyland, T.G. and Hager, D. (1985) Sonography of the liver, gallbladder and spleen. *Veterinary Clinics of North America: Small Animal Practice*, **15**, 1123–1148.

Nyland, T.G. and Park, R.D. (1983) Hepatic ultrasonography in the dog. *Veterinary Radiology*, **24**, 74–84.

Wrigley, R.H., Konde, L.J., Park, R.D. and Lebel, J.L. (1987) Ultrasonographic diagnosis of portocaval shunts in young dogs. *Journal of the American Veterinary Medical Association*, **191**, 421–424.

Wrigley, R.H., Konde, L.J., Park, R.D. and Lebel, J.L. (1988) Ultrasonographic features of splenic lymphosarcoma in dogs: 12 cases (1980–1986). *Journal of the American Veterinary Medical Association*, **193**, 1565–1568.

Wrigley, R.H., Park, R.D., Konde, L.J. and Lebel, J.L. (1988) Ultrasonic features of splenic haemangiosarcomas in dogs: 18 cases (1980–1986). *Journal of the American Veterinary Medical Association*, **192**, 1113–117.

3/Imaging of the Urinary Tract

The kidney

Imaging procedure

The kidneys are easiest to image from the flanks. The animal is placed on its side with the kidney to be examined uppermost. A small patch of hair should be clipped below the sublumbar muscles just behind the last rib on the left and over the last two intercostal spaces on the right. After routine skin preparation and liberal application of acoustic gel, the transducer is placed perpendicular to the skin of the clipped area (Fig. 3.1). The kidney is located superficially beneath the abdominal wall on each side.

When the plane of the sound beam lies parallel to the

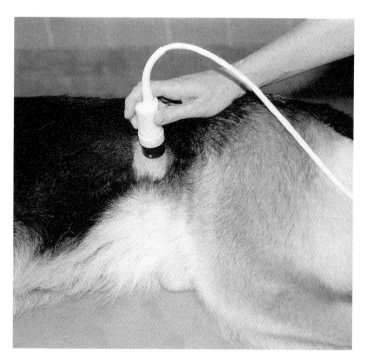

Fig. 3.1 Imaging of the kidney.

lumbar spine a coronal section of the kidney is seen. Fine adjustment should be made to the plane of section until the renal length and width are maximal and the renal pelvis is visible. Rotation of the head of the transducer through 90° allows a transverse section of the kidney to be imaged. A sweep should be made from one pole to the other to ensure that the whole organ is examined. When examination of one kidney is complete, the animal should be turned over and the procedure repeated for the other kidney. The left kidney is often easier to image than the right as it is usually situated behind the last rib. When examining the right kidney, acoustic shadows cast by the ribs may prevent the whole organ being seen at once.

If the animal becomes distressed or struggles when placed on its side, the flank approach may still be used with the animal standing or in sternal recumbency. This can be of particular benefit in cats where minimal restraint often results in cooperative behaviour.

The advantage of the flank approach to imaging of the kidneys is that they are easy to find and image quality is consistently good. Because they lie superficially, minimal tissue penetration is required and a high-frequency transducer (5–10 MHz) may be selected. This allows fine resolution of architectural detail. However, it is important to check the focal depth of the transducer used and if necessary to employ a stand-off to bring the organ within this focal zone.

It is possible to image the kidneys from the ventral abdominal wall. The major disadvantage of this approach is that gas filled bowel is often interposed between the transducer and the kidneys. At best, this results in degradation of image quality and at worst, prevents the kidneys being seen at all. In addition, the depth of penetration required in medium-sized and large dogs limits the frequency of transducer which may be used and thus the image resolution which can be achieved.

Contrast radiography and ultrasound are complementary techniques and thorough renal evaluation may involve both procedures. Each will supply information regarding the shape, size and position of the kidneys. Contrast radiography allows evaluation of renal perfusion and is the more sensitive technique for examination of the renal pelvis and ureters. Ultrasound provides information about the internal renal architecture, even in the absence of renal function. If intravenous urography and ultrasonography are both planned, it may be desirable to perform the examinations at the same time. This is perfectly acceptable as the water-soluble iodinated contrast medium causes no detectable changes in renal architecture or image quality. The resulting osmotic diuresis may cause an increase in renal size but the changes are so small as to be of no practical importance.

Normal appearance

The kidneys of the dog and cat have a similar ultrasonographic appearance (Fig. 3.2). In coronal section the normal kidney is smooth in outline and oval or bean-shaped. A thin echogenic line representing the capsule may be recognized, although this is often less obvious at the curved surface of each pole.

The renal cortex is hypoechoic and finely granular in texture. Echogenicity of the cortex is usually equal to or slightly less than the echogenicity of the liver, and markedly less than the echogenicity of the spleen. As the cranial pole of the right kidney abuts the caudate lobe of the liver, and part of the spleen often lies close to the left kidney, an assessment of relative echogenicity is straightforward.

The renal medulla is virtually anechoic. It lies inside the renal cortex and it is usually divided into sections by diverticula and vessels. Discrete echogenic spots scattered along the corticomedullary junction represent the arcuate vessels.

The renal pelvis is seen as an irregular echogenic mass at the hilus of the kidney. The echogenicity is due to the high fat and fibrous tissue content of this region, and may be so marked that a faint acoustic shadow is cast. It is not normal to see evidence of fluid accumulation (anechoic areas) within the renal pelvis.

The normal proximal ureter is not visible ultrasonographically. However, the renal vein can often be identified running from the renal pelvis to join the caudal vena cava.

Focal parenchymal lesions

Small focal lesions in the kidney parenchyma may be difficult to detect as the normal kidney demonstrates a mixture of echogenicities and textures. In man it is considered that cystic lesions smaller than 1 cm in diameter and solid lesions smaller than 2 cm in diameter cannot be detected reliably using ultrasound. Focal parenchymal lesions may however be detected if they are sufficiently large to cause disruption of the

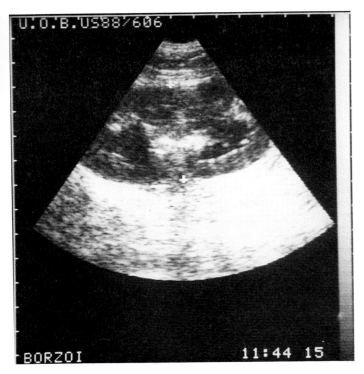

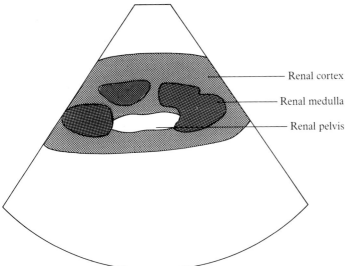

— Renal cortex

— Renal medulla

— Renal pelvis

Fig. 3.2 Normal kidney in a Borzoi. The renal cortex is hypoechoic, the renal medulla is virtually anechoic, and the renal pelvis is echogenic.

normal architecture or distortion of the renal contour. A meticulous search of the entire kidney must always be made to minimize the risk of missing such lesions.

Renal cysts have a characteristic ultrasonographic appearance. They may be single or multiple and may vary greatly in size. Simple cysts are smooth, rounded structures with a well-defined but thin wall and anechoic (fluid) contents. Acoustic enhancement should be visible deep to the cyst itself because of increased sound transmission. Infected or complex cysts may contain septa or debris and may have a rather thicker wall than a simple cyst. If one or more cysts are detected in one kidney, the other kidney should always be examined.

Renal abscesses are uncommon in dogs and cats. The ultrasonographic appearance may vary greatly from ill-defined hypoechoic masses to fluid-filled lesions resembling cysts (Fig. 3.3). Typically an abscess should have a thicker, more irregular wall than a simple cyst, and the fluid often contains some debris — but this is by no means always the case. Consideration of the clinical signs and the results of blood and urine analysis may help clarify the situation.

Focal neoplasms in the kidney may be detected if they are large enough, but small metastatic lesions are often not recognized. The ultrasonographic appearance of primary and secondary tumours in the kidney is variable. Lymphosarcomatous nodules are characteristically homogeneous in texture and echo-poor (Fig. 3.4). They can be differentiated from fluid-filled masses such as cysts, because of the absence of distal acoustic enhancement. Neoplasms of other histological types are variable in echogenicity. Hypervascular tumours tend to be hyperechoic while poorly vascularized lesions of uniform cellularity tend to be hypoechoic. However fine needle aspiration or biopsy is needed to ascertain the histological diagnosis.

Trauma to the kidney can be assessed and monitored using ultrasound. Anechoic collections of fluid associated with subcapsular or perirenal haemorrhage can be readily detected. However, in the early stages it is not possible to distinguish between the accumulation of blood, and leakage of urine resulting from damage to the renal pelvis or ureter. Sequential examination in most cases will show organization and resorption of haemorrhage, while urine accumulations may increase. Alternatively, ultrasound can be used to guide a needle into the fluid, allowing a sample to be withdrawn. Fresh intraparenchymal haemorrhage appears ultrasonographically as echogenic streaks or patches. Sequential examination should demonstrate the resolution of these lesions. Avulsion of the kidney from its arterial supply cannot usually be appreciated ultrasonographically although perirenal haemorrhage will be

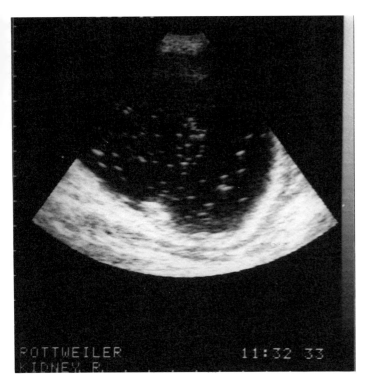

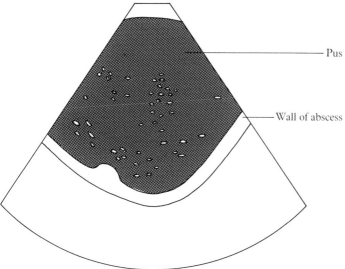

Pus

Wall of abscess

Fig. 3.3 Renal abscess in a
Rottweiler. No normal renal
tissue remains. Small echogenic
particles floating in the pus
represent gas bubbles.

apparent. Contrast radiography is required to make this diagnosis. Complete transection of the kidney occurs rarely but
should be obvious ultrasonographically.

Renal infarcts may occur as a sequel to renal biopsy or in

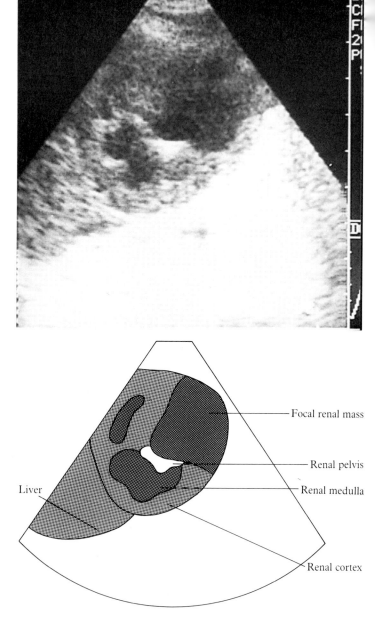

Fig. 3.4 Renal
lymphosarcoma in a Basset
Griffon Vendeen. This is a
transverse section through the
right kidney. Most of the
kidney is architecturally
normal, with cortex, medulla
and pelvis visible. A well-
circumscribed, hypoechoic
wedge in one quadrant
represents the neoplasm.

disease. Fresh infarcts are usually hypoechoic and may bulge
slightly from the surface of the kidney. With scar formation
the infarct becomes more hyperechoic and may cause a de-
pression on the kidney surface.

Diffuse parenchymal disease

Acute diffuse inflammatory diseases of the kidney rarely cause any discernible ultrasonographic changes. Similarly the kidney often looks completely normal in cases of acute renal failure due to hypovolaemia or toxins. It is important to realize therefore that a normal renal sonogram does not rule out renal disease. In acute pyelonephritis an increase in renal size may occur, which is more readily appreciated if the condition is unilateral.

Chronic diffuse parenchymal diseases of the kidney are common in the dog and cat. Glomerular diseases may not cause any ultrasonographic abnormality. However, in many cases of chronic renal disease, irrespective of the aetiology, interstitial fibrosis occurs. This is recognized ultrasonographically by an increase in the echogenicity of the renal cortex (often so marked that it exceeds the hepatic echogenicity). Blurring of the corticomedullary junction and thus of the normal internal architecture often results. The kidneys may be smaller than normal with irregular and indefinite contours and so may be quite difficult to recognise (Fig. 3.5). Although the ultrasonographic changes relate to the severity of the interstitial fibrosis, no definite conclusions should be drawn regarding residual renal function, as this is very variable.

Ultrasound clearly has limitations in the diagnosis of diffuse parenchymal disease, but it may be useful in differentiating acute renal disease from chronic renal disease with acute onset of clinical signs.

Renal neoplasia is often not diagnosed in the dog and cat until it is at an advanced stage. The neoplasm may therefore have replaced all recognizable renal tissue (Fig. 3.6). Such masses are usually mixed in echogenicity with hyperechoic areas representing fibrosis or calcification and hypoechoic regions representing necrosis or haemorrhage. It may not be possible to determine the organ of origin of such a mass other than by confirming the absence of a normal ipsilateral kidney. Diffuse infiltrative neoplasms may cause symmetrical renal enlargement without disturbance of the internal architecture.

Persistent hypercalcaemia in the dog may occur in association with a number of neoplasms (e.g. lymphosarcoma, anal sac adenocarcinoma, multiple myeloma). It may also occur less commonly due to primary hyperparathyroidism. Calcium is a potent nephrotoxin and elevated serum calcium levels will eventually cause irreversible renal damage. The deposition

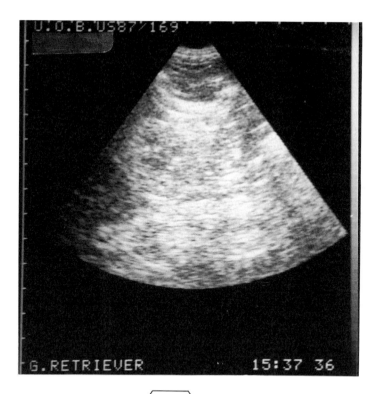

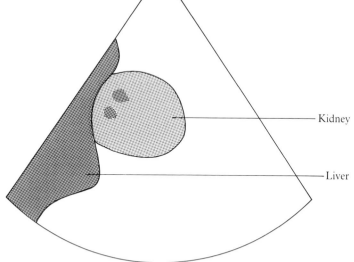

Fig. 3.5 Chronic renal disease in a Golden Retriever. The right kidney is very poorly defined, shrunken and irregular, with little recognizable architecture. Note that the renal cortex is more echogenic than the liver.

of calcium in the renal parenchyma may be detected ultrasonographically. The renal cortex may show a mild to moderate increase in echogenicity. A more striking feature is the presence of a thin, continuous echogenic line at the corticomedullary

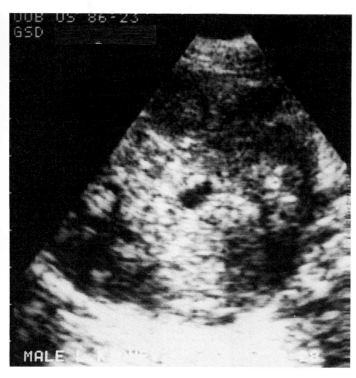

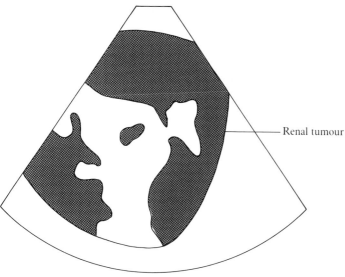

Renal tumour

Fig. 3.6 Primary renal sarcoma in a German Shepherd Dog. The mass is heterogeneous and replaces all normal kidney tissue.

junction, representing heavy calcium deposition at this site (Fig. 3.7). Such an ultrasonographic appearance in the presence of elevated serum calcium levels suggests that renal damage is already extensive.

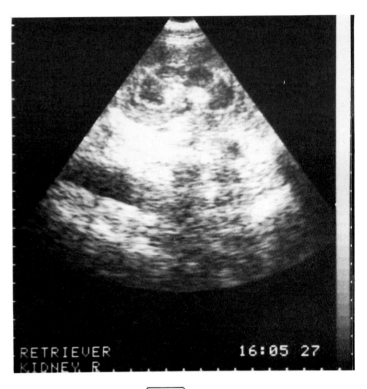

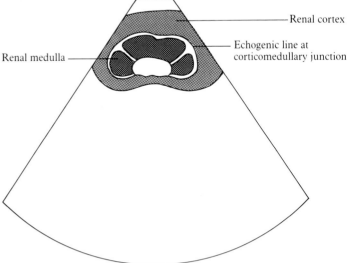

Renal cortex

Echogenic line at
corticomedullary junction

Renal medulla

Fig. 3.7 Hypercalcaemic
nephropathy in a Golden
Retriever. The renal cortex is
increased in echogenicity and
there is a continuous echogenic
line at the corticomedullary
junction.

The collecting system

The commonest abnormality of the collecting system in the
dog and cat is dilation of the renal pelvis and/or ureter. This
may occur as a sequel to obstruction or ascending infection,

and is perhaps most commonly seen in association with ureteral ectopia. Mild cases of hydronephrosis can be difficult to detect ultrasonographically. Early ultrasonographic changes are restricted to scattering of the normal pelvic echoes to form an echogenic ring or horseshoe with an anechoic centre. It is helpful if this anechoic centre can be shown to be continuous with a distended fluid-filled ureter. In mild or moderate hydronephrosis, normal renal parenchyma can be recognized surrounding the distended pelvis.

In more severe cases of hydronephrosis the distended fluid-filled pelvis becomes more obvious and the normal strong echoes of the peripelvic fat and fibrous tissue may be lost completely (Fig. 3.8). The surrounding parenchyma becomes compressed and loses its normal architecture. Eventually the kidney may become a fluid-filled sac with only a thin outer rind. In most severe cases the distended fluid-filled ureter can be detected although it often follows a very tortuous course.

If infection supervenes (pyonephrosis) the fluid within the renal pelvis generally contains debris which settles in the dependent regions.

Renal calculi are readily detected by ultrasonography. Calculi, irrespective of their mineral composition, appear as strongly echogenic specks or lines which cast clear acoustic shadows (Fig. 3.9). The calculus may be localized to the renal parenchyma, the pelvis or proximal ureter. Stones in the middle and distal parts of the ureter are difficult to detect unless there is significant ureteral dilation. Ultrasound is thus a useful technique for the detection of both radiodense and radiolucent calculi, although it is necessary to examine each kidney thoroughly to avoid missing small foci. If medical treatment is used, ultrasound is a safe and non-invasive method of monitoring the dissolution of calculi.

Occasionally an irregular hypoechoic soft tissue mass may be seen within a distended renal pelvis. This may be a neoplasm involving the collecting system, or more commonly a blood clot. The appearance of a blood clot will usually vary with the position of the animal and at subsequent examinations and can thus be differentiated from a soft-tissue mass.

The bladder

Imaging procedure

The bladder is most easily recognized and examined when it is full. Ultrasonographic examination of the bladder should

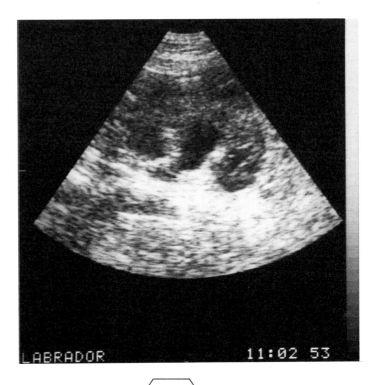

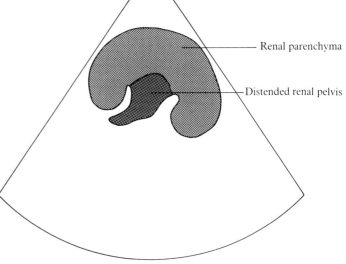

Renal parenchyma

Distended renal pelvis

Fig. 3.8 Hydronephrosis in a
Labrador. The distended,
fluid-filled renal pelvis is clearly
seen. Note the poor
architectural detail and slightly
irregular outline which are due
to associated chronic
pyelonephritis.

therefore ideally be performed before catheterization and contrast radiography. Water-soluble iodinated contrast medium
does not interfere with image quality, but the introduction of
air for pneumocystography or double-contrast cystography
will preclude adequate visualization of the bladder.

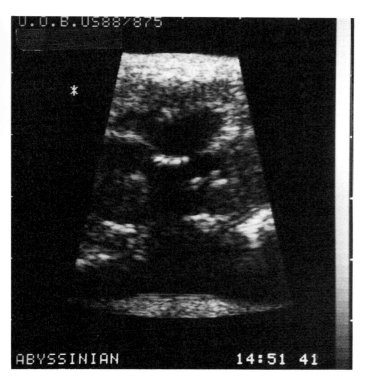

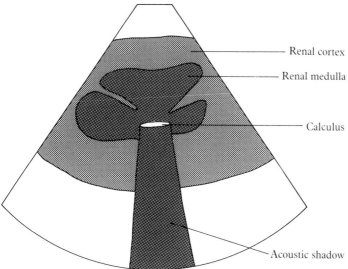

- Renal cortex
- Renal medulla
- Calculus
- Acoustic shadow

Fig. 3.9 Renal calculus in an Abyssinian cat. The calculus is strongly echogenic and casts a clear acoustic shadow.

The animal may be examined standing or in dorsal or lateral recumbency. A small area of hair is clipped between the pubic brim and umbilicus in the midline in the cat or bitch and to one side of the prepuce in the dog. After routine skin preparation the transducer is placed perpendicular to the skin. Once the bladder has been located, it should be imaged in transverse section from the apex to the neck. A longitudinal section should then be taken and a sweep of the transducer made from side to side to ensure that the whole organ is examined.

The bladder is a superficial structure, and since it is fluid filled, little attenuation of the sound beam occurs. Thus the gain settings should be fairly low.

Normal appearance

The normal full bladder in the dog and cat is well-circum-scribed and smooth in outline (Fig. 3.10). The bladder wall is thin and the component layers cannot usually be differentiated unless a high-frequency transducer is used. If the bladder contains only a small amount of urine, the wall naturally appears thicker. The urine within the bladder is usually echolucent so distal acoustic enhancement should be apparent. Occasionally a sediment is visible within the bladder lumen. This shifts to the dependent portion of the bladder if the position of the animal is altered.

It is important to be aware of image artefacts which may be caused by the colon. A full colon may impinge on the bladder, causing distortion of its contour and mimicking a mural mass (Fig.3. 11). Mineral fragments in the colon cast strong acoustic shadows and may be mistaken for cystic calculi. A careful ultrasonographic examination coupled with abdominal pal-pation will usually allow differentiation of colon artefacts and bladder lesions.

The bladder lumen

The presence of a sediment in the bladder lumen which shifts as the position of the animal changes may be a normal finding. However, it may also imply the presence of urinary tract infection (Fig. 3.12). In the cat, sediment of gravel in the bladder usually suggests a diagnosis of urolithiasis.

Cystic calculi are easily detected using ultrasound. Calculi, irrespective of their mineral composition, are strongly echo-genic and cast clear acoustic shadows (Fig. 3.13). Calculi which are floating free in the lumen of the bladder may be differentiated from calcification of mural lesions by demon-strating that they shift as the animal changes its position.

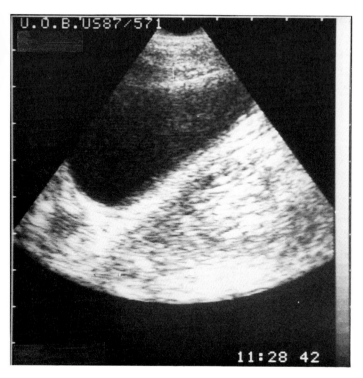

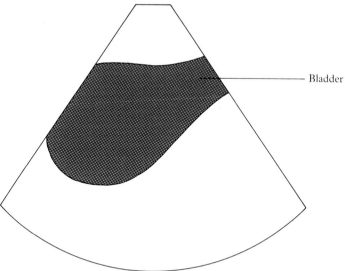

Bladder

Fig. 3.10 Normal bladder in a Boxer.

Stones may also occasionally be detected within the prostatic urethra.

Blood clots in the urine may arise from cystic or renal lesions. They are usually irregular in shape and hypoechoic

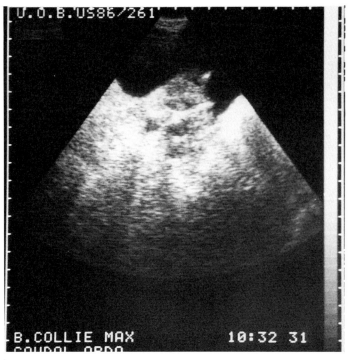

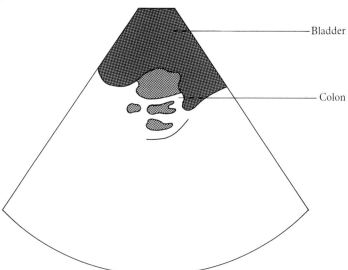

Fig. 3.11 Normal bladder in a Border Collie. The colon is full of faeces and indents the bladder, giving the false impression of a mural mass.

and once again will move as the animal changes its position. If a blood clot is adherent to the bladder wall it may not be possible to differentiate it from a soft-tissue mass.

If the bladder is overstretched for any length of time or

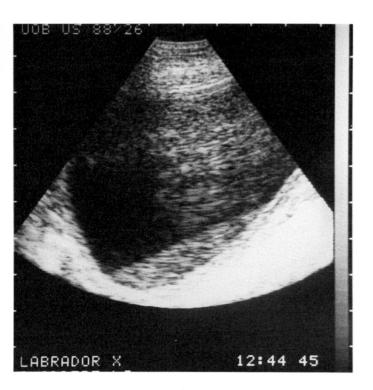

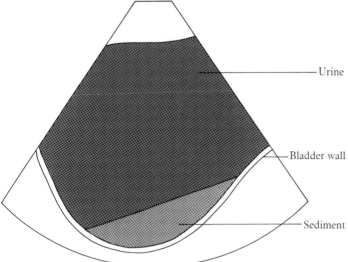

Urine

Bladder wall

Sediment

Fig. 3.12 Sediment in the bladder associated with chronic urinary tract infection in a cross-breed dog. The sediment will shift as the position of the dog is changed.

severely inflamed, sloughing of the mucosa into the bladder lumen may occur. This can be detected ultrasonographically. A linear echogenicity may be seen lifting from the internal aspect of the bladder wall. After total separation has occurred,

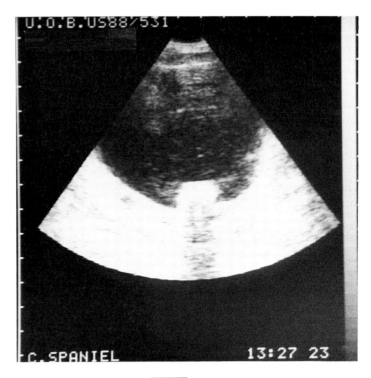

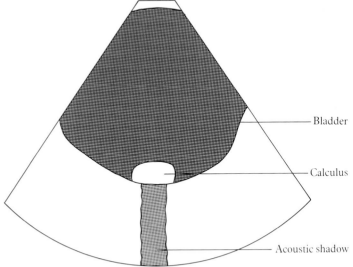

Bladder

Calculus

Acoustic shadow

Fig. 3.13 Cystic calculus in a Cocker Spaniel. The highly echogenic calculus sits in the dependent portion of the bladder. A faint acoustic shadow is seen.

an amorphous hypoechoic mass may be detected floating freely within the bladder lumen.

The bladder wall

Inflammatory thickening of the bladder wall may be difficult to detect ultrasonographically unless it is very severe. The most common site for inflammatory lesions is the cranioventral part of the bladder wall. There may be associated sediment and even blood clots and/or calculi in the urine.

Neoplastic lesions of the bladder wall may be detected if they are large enough. In some cases a clear mural mass projecting into the lumen is seen (Fig. 3.14), while in other cases a diffuse irregular thickening of the wall is apparent. Associated blood clots adherent to the wall or free in the lumen may be seen. If surgery is contemplated, it is important to try to assess the site of the lesion in relation to the bladder neck and the points of entry of the ureters. The size of the mass and whether it is pedunculated or broad-based should also be noted. It is difficult to evaluate the degree of mural and extra mural invasion unless a high-frequency transducer is used (7.5 MHz or above).

Although it is preferable to evaluate the bladder wall when the bladder is distended, many animals with inflammatory or neoplastic lesions of the bladder wall show increased frequency of urination. In such cases it may be necessary to put fluid into the bladder under anaesthesia to achieve adequate bladder distension. The fluid may be water-soluble iodinated contrast medium if the procedure is to be combined with contrast radiography, or saline. In those cases where a neoplasm is obstructing urine outflow the bladder may be very distended already.

Rupture of the bladder cannot be diagnosed with any certainty by ultrasound. The presence of free abdominal fluid and the absence of a recognizable bladder is suggestive of bladder rupture but not diagnostic. Similarly, the identification of an apparently normal bladder does not preclude a small leak or avulsion of the bladder from the urethra.

In cases of ureteral ectopia and hydroureter the distended ureter may be seen running across the dorsal surface and neck of the bladder. If a ureterocoele is present, an intramural elliptical fluid-filled swelling may be imaged near the bladder neck.

The prostate

Imaging procedure

Prostatic disease is rare in the cat and there are few indications for the ultrasonographic examination of this organ.

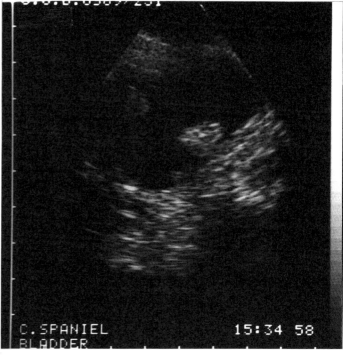

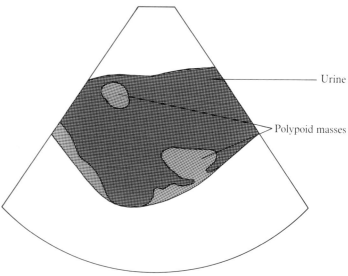

Urine

Polypoid masses

Fig. 3.14 Polypoid masses arising from the bladder wall in a Cocker Spaniel. Mural masses remain fixed even when the position of the dog is changed.

The imaging technique described applies to the dog but may if necessary be used for the cat.

Ultrasonographic examination of the prostate gland may be performed by rectal or transabdominal routes. The rectal approach has the advantage of allowing the prostate to be imaged even when it lies in an intrapelvic position, but a transducer designed specifically for rectal work is necessary. A transabdominal approach is in most instances satisfactory, and no specialized transducer is required.

The examination should be performed with the bladder moderately distended. A full bladder acts as an easily recognizable landmark and displaces gas-filled small intestine from the caudal abdomen. The dog should be placed in dorsal or lateral recumbency and a small area of hair clipped to one side of the prepuce just in front of the pubic brim. After routine skin preparation the transducer should be placed perpendicular to the skin surface with the plane of the beam approximately parallel to the prepuce. Once the bladder has been identified, it is possible to move caudally towards the neck of the bladder and thence to the prostate. If the prostate lies partly or wholly within the pelvic canal, it may be necessary to angle the transducer caudally under the pubic rim (Fig. 3.15). Alternatively, a gloved finger may be placed per rectum and the prostate pushed gently forward. Occasionally, in immature dogs or dogs which have been neutered at a young age, it may prove impossible to image the prostate, but in such cases prostatic disease is unlikely.

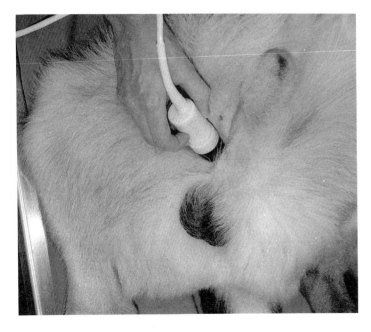

Fig. 3.15 Imaging of the prostate.

Once the prostate has been identified in longitudinal section, a sweep from side to side should be made. The transducer should then be rotated through 90° to achieve a transverse section and a sweep made from one end of the gland to the other. In this way a thorough examination of the entire gland can be made. It may on occasions be helpful to place an air- or fluid-filled urethral catheter *in situ* to enable an assessment of prostatic symmetry to be made.

Normal appearance

The normal prostate in the dog is smooth in outline and fairly well-circumscribed (Fig. 3.16). It varies in shape from almost spherical to clearly bilobed or pear-shaped. The prostatic parenchyma is normally moderately echoic with a coarse but even texture throughout. Linear echogenic streaks may be detected running longitudinally through the middle of the gland. This is the 'hilar echo' and is thought to represent periurethral fibrous tissue. The prostatic urethra itself is not usually visible in the conscious dog, but during general anaesthesia a narrow fluid-filled urethra is sometimes seen running through the prostate.

Variations in the size and ultrasonographic appearance of the normal prostate according to age and history of neutering have not yet been defined.

Focal parenchymal lesions

Focal disturbances in the normal even echotexture of the prostate should be carefully evaluated. The number of lesions, their size and shape, the clarity of their outline and their echogenicity should all be noted. It is also important to determine whether lesions are intra- or paraprostatic.

The commonest focal lesions identified on ultrasonographic examination of the prostate are intraprostatic cysts. Small cysts (less than 1 cm in diameter) with a smooth, well-defined wall and fluid contents are generally of little clinical significance and probably represent accumulation of prostatic secretions (Fig. 3.17). Larger cysts may cause asymmetrical prostatic enlargement. The wall may be thick and irregular, and the centre may be septated or contain debris. Prostatic abscesses (Fig. 3.18) or tumours with a cystic component may have an identical ultrasonographic appearance, so needle as-

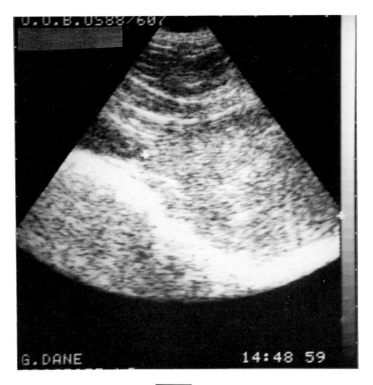

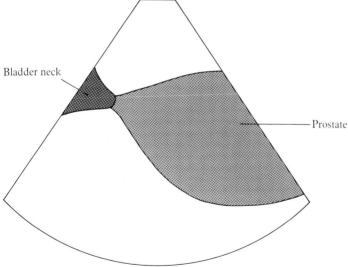

Fig.3.16 Normal prostate in an entire Great Dane. The gland is smooth in outline, symmetrical in shape, and even in texture.

piration of the contents may be required for a definitive diagnosis.

In cases of prostatic haemorrhage, ultrasonographic examination of the prostate is often unrewarding. Although haema-

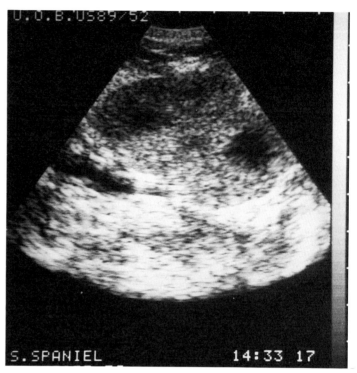

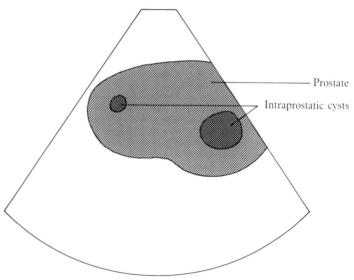

Fig. 3.17 Intraprostatic cysts in a Springer Spaniel. This is a transverse section through the prostate, showing a small cyst in each lobe.

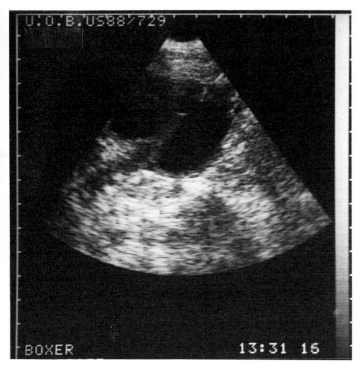

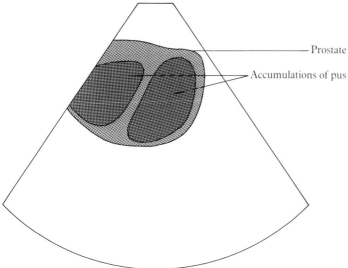

Fig. 3.18 Prostatic abscess in a Boxer. This transverse section through the prostate reveals two large, fluid-filled cavities. Aspiration of the fluid showed it to be pus.

tomata or haematocysts have been reported, in many instances the prostate appears ultrasonographically normal.

Diffuse parenchymal disease

Benign prostatic hypertrophy is a common condition in entire male dogs. The prostate often appears enlarged but remains smooth in outline and a normal shape. The echotexture is still even but a slight overall increase in echogenicity has been noted by some authors. The hilar echo is thought to become less obvious, either as a result of the overall increase in echogenicity or because of compression. In practical terms, it is difficult to differentiate a normal prostate and a hypertrophied prostate ultrasonographically, except on the basis of size.

In acute prostatitis, the prostate is usually enlarged (Fig. 3.19). In severe cases a distinctly mottled texture is seen with an overall decrease in echogenicity. The hypoechoic patches seen presumably represent areas of haemorrhage, necrosis or abscess formation. With extension of inflammatory changes into the periprostatic tissues, the outline of the prostate may become rather poorly defined.

Chronic prostatitis may also result in a patchy density, but in this instance the overall impression is of an increase in echogenicity. Hyperechoic areas probably represent fibrosis or calcification. The gland is of variable size in such cases but may be irregular in outline.

Prostatic tumours in the dog are usually not diagnosed until they reach a relatively advanced stage. Thus, localized nodules within otherwise normal prostatic parenchyma, as described in man, are not usually identified. Instead a moderately enlarged prostate is seen, often with irregular and indistinct margins. The echotexture is patchy with an overall increase in echogenicity (Fig. 3.20). From this description it is apparent that it is difficult to differentiate prostatic neoplasia and chronic prostatitis by ultrasonography alone. It has been suggested that focal mineralization with acoustic shadowing is more suggestive of neoplasia than chronic prostatitis in the dog. The demonstration of enlarged sublumbar lymph nodes is more likely in neoplasia but may also occur in cases of chronic infection. Biopsy is therefore usually required for a definitive diagnosis.

Paraprostatic disease

Paraprostatic cysts vary greatly in size, shape and position.

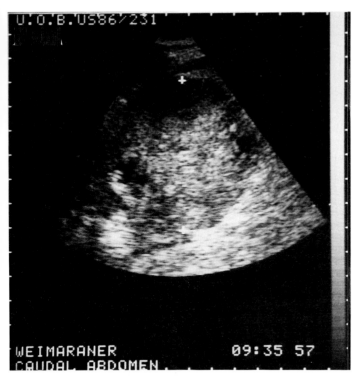

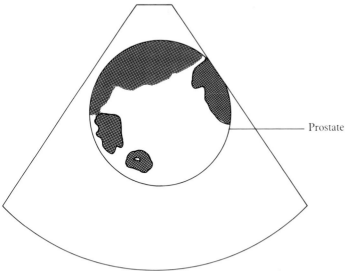

Prostate

Fig. 3.19 Acute prostatitis in a Weimaraner. The parenchymal texture is very heterogeneous, because of the severe inflammatory changes. The outline of the prostate is poorly defined owing to extension of the inflammatory process into the periprostatic tissues.

They are usually well-circumscribed with thin smooth walls and fluid contents. Internal septa are common, and in some cysts the presence of multiple septa gives the appearance of a honeycomb or a sponge (Fig. 3.21). A variable amount

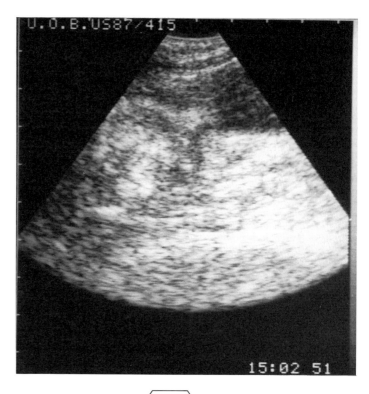

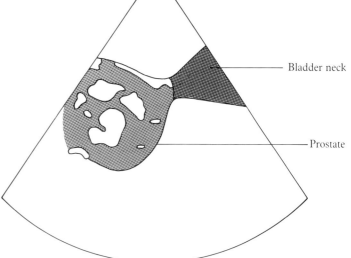

Fig. 3.20 Prostatic carcinoma in a Border Collie. The prostate is poorly defined, and contains multiple, irregular echogenic patches.

of solid tissue is present. Mineralization of the wall of prostatic cysts is not uncommon, and will be recognized ultrasonographically by the presence of acoustic shadowing. The prostate should normally be identifiable as a separate structure.

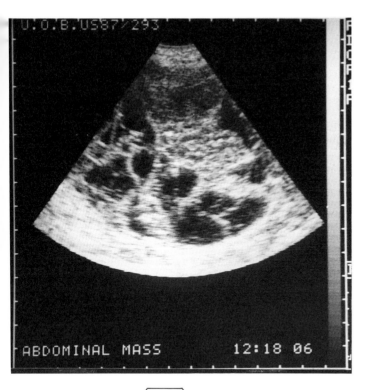

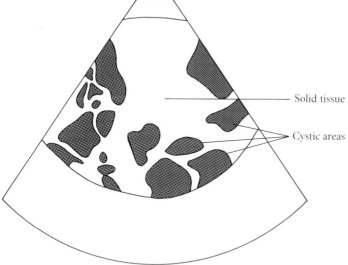

Solid tissue

Cystic areas

Fig. 3.21 Paraprostatic cyst in a cross-breed dog. This cyst has a fairly large component of solid tissue, with multiple cystic spaces giving the appearance of a honeycomb.

It is not possible to ascertain ultrasonographically whether such cysts have a neoplastic component or not. Biopsy of the cyst wall during surgery is usually necessary to determine this.

In cases of perineal rupture, either the bladder or a paraprostatic cyst may pass caudally into the perineum. Ultrasonography of the perineal swelling will confirm the presence of a large fluid-filled structure. If internal septa are present the structure can be identified as a paraprostatic cyst. If the structure is smooth in outline with no divisions it may be a simple cyst or the bladder, and contrast urethrocystography will be needed to clarify the situation.

Further reading

Barr, F.J., Patteson, M.W., Lucke, V.M. and Gibbs, C. (1989) Hypercalcaemic nephropathy in three dogs: sonographic appearance. *Veterinary Radiology*, **30**, 169–173.

Cartee, R.E. and Rowles, T. (1983) Transabdominal sonographic evaluation of the canine prostate. *Veterinary Radiology*, **24**, 156–164.

Cartee, R.E., Selcer, B.A. and Patton, C.S. (1980) Ultrasonographic diagnosis of renal disease in small animals. *Journal of the American Veterinary Medical Association*, **176**, p. 426.

Feeney, D.A., Johnston, G.R. and Klausner, J.S. (1985) Two-dimensional gray-scale ultrasonography: application in canine prostatic disease. *Veterinary Clinics of North America: Small Animal Practice*. Diagnostic Ultrasound. **15**, 1159–1176.

Feeney, D.A., Johnston, G.R., Klausner, J.S., Perman, V., Leininger, J.R. and Tomlinson, M.J. (1987) Canine prostatic disease—comparison of ultrasonographic appearance with morphologic and microbiologic findings: 30 cases (1981–1985). *Journal of the American Veterinary Medical Association*, **190**, 1027–1034.

Johnston, G.R., Walker, P.A. and Feeney, D.A. (1986) Radiographic and ultrasonographic features of uroliths and other urinary tract filling defects. *Veterinary Clinics of North America: Small Animal Practice*. Canine Urolithiasis. **16**, 261–292.

Konde, L.J. (1985) Sonography of the kidney. *Veterinary Clinics of North America: Small Animal Practice* Diagnostic Ultrasound. **15**, 1149–1158.

Konde, L.J., Park, R.D., Wrigley, R.H. and Lebel J.L. (1986) Comparison of radiography and ultrasonography in the evaluation of renal lesions in the dog. *Journal of the American Veterinary Medical Association*, **188**, 1420–1425.

Konde, L.J., Wrigley, R.H., Park, R.D. and Lebel, J.L. (1984) Ultrasonographic anatomy of the normal canine kidney. *Veterinary Radiology*, **25**, 173–178.

Konde, L.J., Wrigley, R.H., Park, R.D. and Lebel, J.L. (1985) Sonographic appearance of renal neoplasia in the dog. *Veterinary Radiology*. **26**, 74–81.

Walter, P.A., Feeney, D.A., Johnston, G.R. and Fletcher, T.F. (1987) Feline renal ultrasonography: quantitative analyses of imaged anatomy. *American Journal of Veterinary Research*, **48**, 596–599.

Walter, P.A., Feeney, D.A., Johnston, G.R. and O'Leary, T.P. (1987) Ultrasonographic evaluation of renal parenchymal disease in dogs: 32 cases (1981–1986). *Journal of the American Veterinary Medical Association*, **191**, 999–1007.

Walter, P.A., Johnston, G.R., Feeney, D.A. and O'Brien, T.D. (1987)

Renal ultrasonography in healthy cats. *American Journal of Veterinary Research*, **48**, 600–607.

Walter, P.A., Johnston, D.R., Feeney, D.A. and O'Brien, T.D. (1988) Applications of ultrasonography in the diagnosis of parenchymal kidney disease in cats: 24 cases (1981–1986) *Journal of the American Veterinary Medical Association*, **192**, 92–98.

4/Imaging of the Reproductive Tract

The uterus

Imaging procedure

The uterus is most easily examined with the animal in dorsal or lateral recumbency, but it is also possible to image the uterus with the animal standing. Some cats prefer to be supported in an upright position with their front legs held up and their back legs on the table. An area of hair should be clipped from the umbilicus to the pubis, extending several centimetres to each side of the midline. Particular care needs to be taken when clipping this area if mammary development is present. After routine skin preparation, the transducer should be placed perpendicular to the skin just cranial to the pubis.

In women the full urinary bladder is used as an acoustic window through which the entire uterus can be imaged. The dog and cat have a long bicornuate uterus so this is not possible. Nevertheless, the full bladder acts as a useful landmark. The transducer should be moved cranially until the bladder is identified.

The cervix, uterine body and bifurcation are usually located dorsal to the bladder and ventral to the colon. If the colon is very full of faeces, it is worth giving the animal the opportunity to defaecate before repeating the examination. If a tubular structure is identified dorsal to the bladder, it should be followed cranially to its bifurcation in order to confirm that the structure seen is uterus rather than bowel. A search should also be made cranial to the bladder for the uterine horns.

Normal appearance of the nongravid uterus

The normal nongravid uterus in the dog and cat is often not visible ultrasonographically. In the dog, an ovoid hypoechoic mass representing the cervix may sometimes be identified lying between the dorsal wall of the bladder and the descending colon (Fig. 4.1). A narrow hypoechoic tubular structure can occasionally be followed cranially until it divides into two. The uterine horns cranial to the bladder cannot be identified

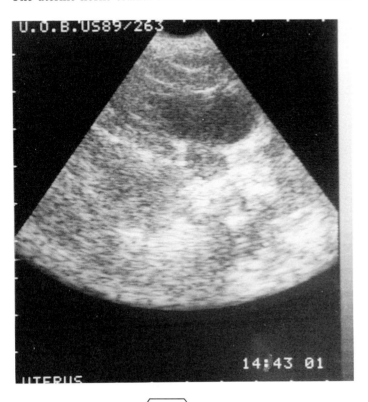

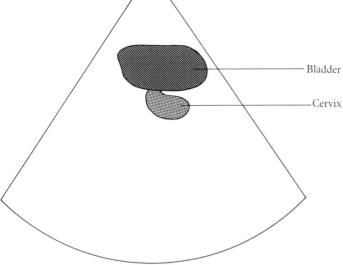

Fig. 4.1 Normal cervix in a Keeshond. This is a transverse section through the bladder and cervix.

with certainty as they cannot be distinguished from bowel loops.

Normal appearance of the gravid uterus

In the bitch, gestational sacs containing fetal tissue suspended in amniotic fluid are first consistently seen between days 24 and 28 of gestation. Before this time it may not be possible to differentiate the uterus from fluid-filled bowel loops. As a rule of thumb, if fetal structures can be confidently identified before day 28, a positive diagnosis of pregnancy can be made. However, a negative result should not be confirmed until 28 days after the last mating.

The gestational sacs of early pregnancy are rounded, well-circumscribed masses containing fluid which should be completely echo-free. The uterine wall/placenta may be identified forming a hypoechoic ring around the sac. Within the fluid, the fetus is seen as an echogenic, comma-shaped structure. Depending on the frequency of the transducer used and therefore the resolution of structures achieved, the fetal membranes may also be recognized as linear echogenicities within the fluid (Fig. 4.2). The size and development of the fetus at this stage is very variable, probably because of discrepancies between the time of mating and the time of conception. Bitches have been reported to conceive when mated as early as 11 days before or as late as 3 days after oocyte maturation.

A small but persistent and regular flickering can often be detected within the fetal tissue from 28 days onwards. This is the fetal heart which usually beats at 120–140 beats/per min. Generalized fetal movements can also be seen at this early stage, allowing assessment of fetal viability as well as pregnancy diagnosis.

Between days 34 and 37 of gestation (and sometimes earlier) a distinct fetal head and body can be identified (Fig. 4.3). Head-turning and swimming movements are seen. Between days 38 and 45, organ development can be recognized ultrasonographically (Fig. 4.4). The heart becomes easier to see — it is a rounded anechoic structure with echogenic septa representing chamber divisions and valves. The beating of the fetal heart is usually obvious. The lungs are obviously not air-filled in the fetus, and appear moderately echoic. The fetal liver is hypoechoic and occupies a large part of the abdomen. The stomach usually contains amniotic fluid and so is visible as a rounded anechoic structure lying close to or apparently

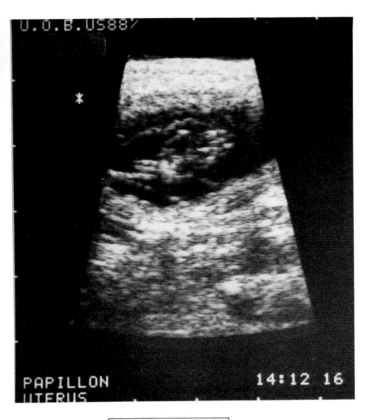

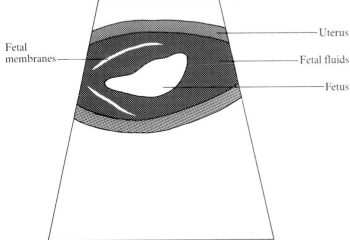

Fetal membranes

Uterus

Fetal fluids

Fetus

Fig. 4.2 Normal pregnancy of 24–28 days gestation in a Papillon. A high-frequency transducer (10 MHz) has been used, allowing fine detail of the fetus and fetal membranes to be seen. The uterine wall can also be identified.

within the liver. The urinary bladder is also anechoic but is situated caudally. The vertebrae are hyperechoic areas arranged in a segmented pattern along the length of the body. The other skeletal structures are similarly hyperechoic. As skeletal

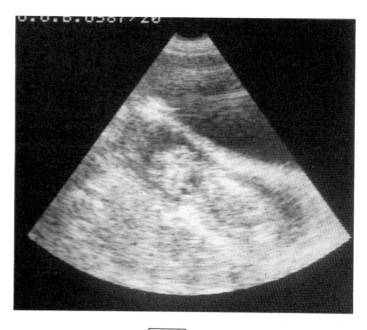

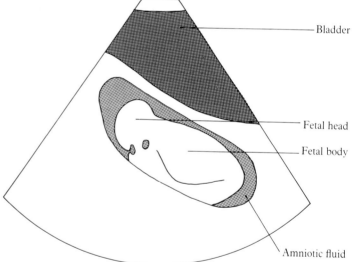

Bladder

Fetal head

Fetal body

Amniotic fluid

Fig. 4.3 Normal pregnancy of about 30 days gestation in a Briard. The head and body of the fetus can be recognized.

mineralization progresses, acoustic shadowing becomes obvious. Although the fetal organs can be identified and examined using ultrasound, developmental anomalies are only occasionally detected. Further experience of ultrasound may allow more fetal abnormalities to be recognized *in utero*, although the practical value of this in a multiple pregnancy with the option of euthanasia of abnormal fetuses at birth may be limited.

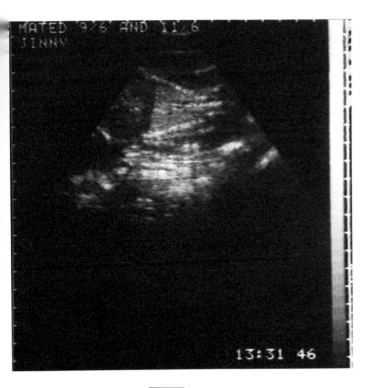

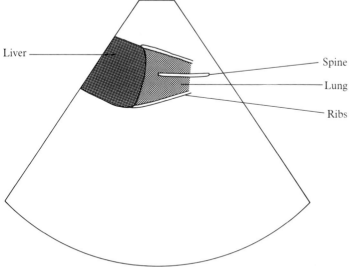

Fig. 4.4 Normal pregnancy of about 50 days gestation in a Boxer. Details of the fetal organs can be recognized at this stage.

Normal fetal dimensions at different stages of gestation have been measured in the dog. The results of one study show that the canine fetus grows rapidly in body diameter between the fourth and fifth week of gestation. About 1 week later it grows rapidly in body length and head diameter. One week later the body diameter accelerates again. Thus although there is considerable variation in absolute measurements at the same stage of gestation, even within a litter, the pattern of growth can be used if necessary to assess the progression of a pregnancy.

The ultrasonographic appearance of the gravid uterus in the cat is similar to that described in the dog, but pregnancy diagnosis may be possible at an earlier stage of gestation.

Ultrasonographic determination of fetal numbers in the dog and cat is difficult. Counting is easiest at 28–35 days gestation when the fetuses are still small. When the fetuses are too large to be imaged in their entirety, only sections of the fetal bodies are seen and counting can be very confusing. However, even if a systematic search of the abdomen is made at the optimum time, it is difficult to be certain that the same fetus has not been counted more than once or one excluded. Litters of five or under can be counted with more accuracy than larger litters, but it is probably wise to limit predictions to a 'large' or 'small' litter size!

Abnormalities of the uterus

During pregnancy, fetal distress and death may be detected ultrasonographically. A diminution of generalized fetal activity and slowing of the fetal heart rate is indicative of fetal distress. If a careful and systematic examination of the fetus fails to show cardiac activity then fetal death is likely. This is important clinical information which may help decide whether veterinary intervention is indicated. If fetal death is long-standing, gas may accumulate within the uterus and/or within the fetus. This can be detected ultrasonographically as echogenic spots or streaks which cast acoustic shadows, but care must be taken to differentiate gas from the normal skeletal structures which also cast acoustic shadows. As fetal maceration proceeds, recognizable fetal structure is lost and irregular echogenic accumulations of debris within a fluid-filled uterine lumen are seen.

Therefore, ultrasound is useful for fetal monitoring in the overdue bitch or queen, and during a prolonged parturition. It may also confirm the absence of viable fetuses during or after spontaneous abortion (Fig. 4.5). Uterine involution postpartum can also be checked if necessary.

Pyometritis is probably the commonest uterine disorder

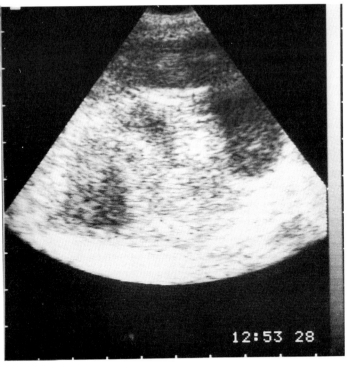

12:53 28

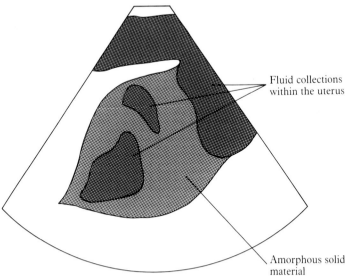

Fluid collections
within the uterus

Amorphous solid
material

Fig. 4.5 Spontaneous
abortion in a German Short-
Haired Pointer. This bitch had
been scanned a week previously
and viable fetuses seen. Now
irregular fluid collections and
amorphous debris can be seen
in the uterus, but no
recognizable fetal structure.

diagnosed in the dog and cat. Ultrasound is a quick and
simple means of diagnosis. Distended, fluid-filled uterine horns
and body may be identified cranial and dorsal to the bladder
(Fig. 4.6). Often the horns are so distended that they cannot

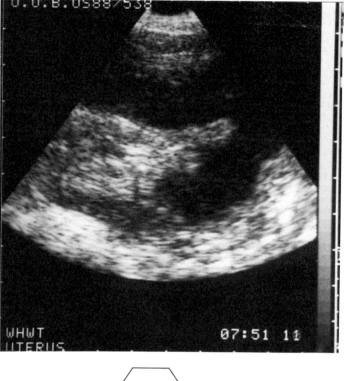

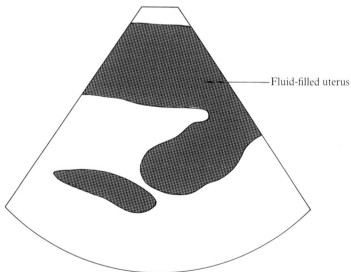

Fluid-filled uterus

Fig. 4.6 Pyometra in a West Highland White Terrier. A distended, fluid-filled uterine horn is visible.

be mistaken for normal fluid-filled bowel loops. If less marked enlargement is present, the horns must be followed caudally to the uterine body dorsal to the bladder to confirm their identity. The absence of peristalsis in the uterus may also help distinguish the uterus from the gastrointestinal tract. The contents of the uterus in pyometritis are of variable ultrasonographic appearance. Most often the contents are fluid and therefore anechoic. In some cases the presence of debris results in echoes within the fluid, but any masses within the lumen are amorphous and quite distinct from the structure of a fetus. It is not possible to differentiate between pyometra and haematometra or hydrometra using ultrasound alone.

Granulomata or abscesses of the uterine stump may be detected ultrasonographically depending on their size. An irregular mass, usually of mixed echogenicity, can be seen lying between the dorsal wall of the bladder and the colon. The appearance of this mass should be less regular and ordered than the smooth oval of the normal cervix. However, failure to detect such a mass does not rule out the diagnosis as the lesion may be small and obscured by bowel loops.

Uterine tumours are uncommon. Ultrasonographically, a mass may be found in the caudal abdomen. The ultrasonographic appearance is likely to vary according to the tumour type and the presence of haemorrhage or necrosis. It may not be possible to be certain that the mass is uterine in origin unless there is associated fluid distension of the uterus.

The ovary

Imaging procedure

The normal ovaries are difficult to identify in the dog and cat. The ovary is usually located caudal to the ipsilateral kidney. Thus, if the animal is in lateral recumbency, the imaging procedure for the kidney may be followed. Once the kidney is identified, the transducer should be moved caudally to search for the ovary. If the animal is examined in a standing position, the ovaries tend to drop ventrally, suspended by the mesovarium. It is helpful to identify the kidney first and then to move caudally and ventrally to search for the ovary.

Abnormally enlarged ovaries may drop to lie in the ventral part of the caudal or mid abdomen, and may therefore be imaged from the ventral abdominal wall. It is difficult to examine normal ovaries from this approach because of interference from intervening bowel loops.

Normal appearance

It may prove impossible to identify the normal ovaries in the dog and cat. When the ovaries are recognized, they are usually smooth in outline and approximately oval in shape. They are moderately hypoechoic and of even echotexture.

There has been a published report of the ultrasonographic detection of follicles within the ovary in the bitch and the disappearance of the follicle at the time of ovulation (Inaba *et al.*, 1984). Theoretically, follicles should have the appearance of a simple cyst with thin, well-defined walls and fluid contents. Other work has indicated that the ultrasonographic appearance of the ovary in the bitch does not alter at the time of ovulation (England and Allen, 1989). The resolving capacity of the transducer used will obviously affect the detail seen in the imaged ovary. Nevertheless, the value of ultrasound in monitoring follicular development and the time of ovulation in the bitch remains unproven at present.

Abnormalities of the ovary

Large polycystic ovaries are usually easily detected. They often fall into the mid or ventral part of the caudal abdomen. An irregular but well-circumscribed mass with thin walls and fluid contents is seen. Multiple septa are visible internally (Fig. 4.7). The presence of solid tissue as well as cysts within the mass is suggestive of neoplasia. However, masses which appear purely cystic may also have a neoplastic component. Histology of the resected ovary is required for a definitive diagnosis.

Ovarian tumours are variable in their ultrasonographic appearance. Clinical signs are often not noticed until the tumour is advanced, so the mass may be quite large. It may be fixed in the dorsal part of the abdomen due to local invasion, or may drop into the mid or ventral parts of the abdomen. Ovarian tumours are usually of mixed echogenicity and may have a cystic component (Fig. 4.8). Free abdominal and/or thoracic fluid may be detected in association with some malignant ovarian tumours.

The testes

Imaging procedure

Testicular disease is uncommon in the cat and indications for the ultrasonographic examination of the feline testicle are therefore limited. The imaging procedure is described with reference to the dog but may be adapted for the cat if necessary.

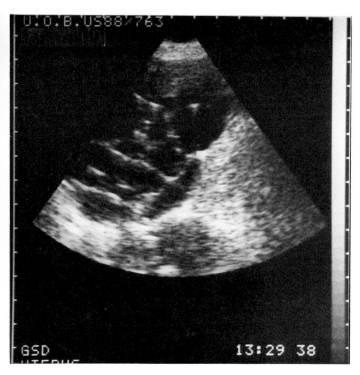

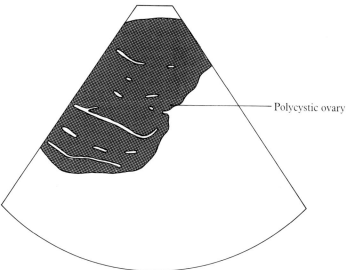

Polycystic ovary

Fig. 4.7 Polycystic ovary in a German Shepherd Dog. A well-defined, fluid-filled mass with multiple septa is seen.

Ultrasonographic examination of the scrotal testicle is straightforward. It is rarely necessary to clip the scrotal area in the dog. Acoustic gel should be applied liberally to the skin and the transducer placed over the testicle. Depending on the

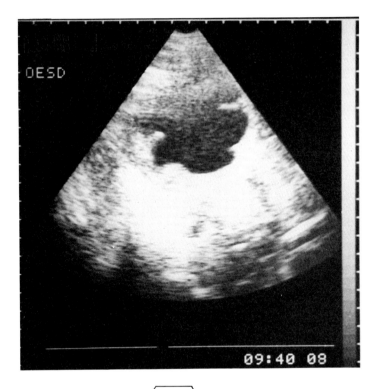

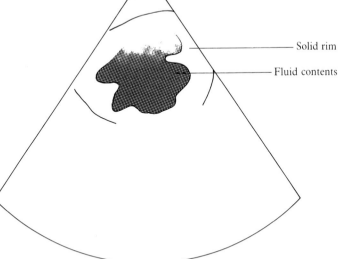

Fig. 4.8 Ovarian tumour in
an Old English Sheepdog. The
image quality here is poor as
the gain has been set too high.
However, a mass with a fluid
centre and a thick, irregular
rind is visible.

size of the transducer used, the testicles may be examined
separately or together. A systematic examination of the entire
testicular parenchyma should be made. The scrotal testicle is
clearly a very superficial structure. Therefore it is preferable

to select a high-frequency transducer to optimize image resolution. It may be necessary to use a stand-off to bring the testicle within the focal zone of the sound beam.

If the testicle is inguinal, it may be palpable. In these cases the transducer can be placed directly over the organ. If it is necessary to search for a non-scrotal testicle, the search should begin in the inguinal region. A systematic search of the region may reveal the testicle. If it does not, an area of skin from the pubis to the umbilicus on the appropriate side of the midline should be clipped and prepared. The abdomen may then be examined. The search should begin just in front of the pubis in the region of the inguinal ring, progress to the region of the bladder, and finally end in the area between the bladder and the ipsilateral kidney. It should be recognized however that an intra-abdominal testicle may be difficult to detect unless it is enlarged.

Normal appearance

The normal testicle is usually well-circumscribed, smooth in outline and oval in shape (Fig. 4.9). A thin echogenic capsule may be apparent. The parenchyma should be finely granular, even in texture, and of moderate echogenicity. An echogenic spot or line in the centre of the organ is quite commonly noticed. The epididymis may be detected adjacent to the testicle. It is coarser in texture than the testicular parenchyma and somewhat irregular in outline.

Abnormalities of the testicle

The most common parenchymal abnormalities of the testicle in the dog are neoplastic. Tumours may be small and difficult to detect by palpation, or they may be large enough to distort the outline of the organ and may replace all recognizable normal testicular tissue. Neoplasms vary in their ultrasonographic appearance. In man, most testicular tumours are homogeneous and of reduced echogenicity compared to the normal parenchyma. However, some neoplasms (notably teratomata) have a very heterogeneous ultrasonographic pattern. Limited experience indicates that the ultrasonographic appearance of testicular tumours in dogs is equally variable and that the tumour type cannot be predicted from the echogenicity and echo-pattern (Fig. 4.10).

Not all focal parenchymal lesions in the testicle are neo-

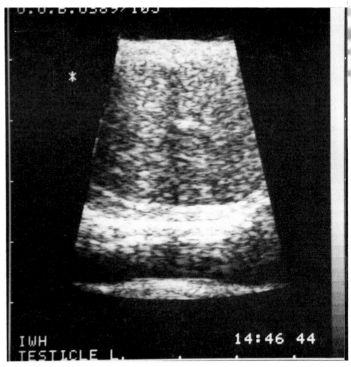

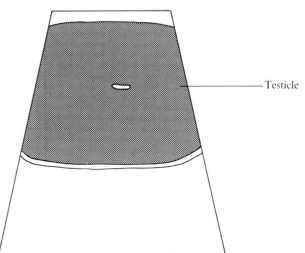

Testicle

Fig. 4.9 Normal testicle in an Irish Wolfhound. The parenchyma is of an even, coarse granularity.

plastic — abscesses, granulomata and haematomata may also occur. Although ultrasound is sensitive in the detection of focal lesions in the testicular parenchyma, it is not possible to differentiate benign and malignant lesions with any certainty.

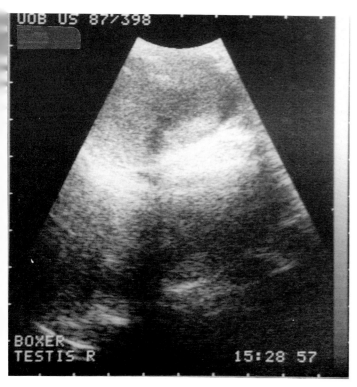

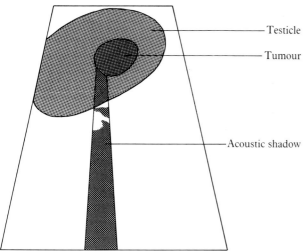

Testicle

Tumour

Acoustic shadow

Fig. 4.10 Testicular tumour in a Boxer. The tumour is shown as a poorly defined, hypoechoic mass within normal testicular parenchyma. A small area of acoustic shadowing is seen, probably arising from a focus of calcification.

Biopsy or histological examination of the excised organ is necessary for a definitive diagnosis.

Ultrasound is useful in allowing differentiation between testicular and extratesticular disease. The accumulation of

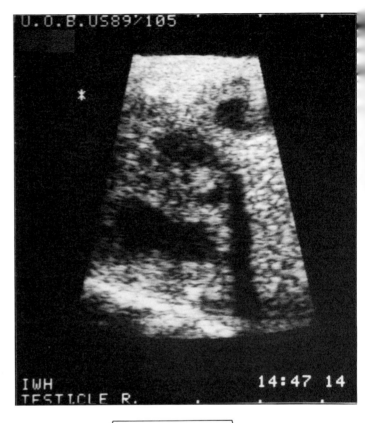

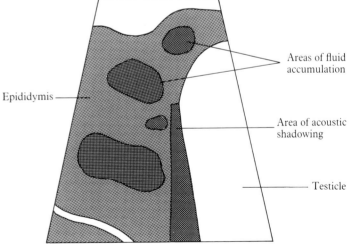

Fig. 4.11 Epididymitis in an Irish Wolfhound. Irregular accumulations of fluid can be seen within the enlarged epididymis. The acoustic shadow is probably due to an area of mineralization. Normal testicular parenchyma is visible adjacent to the epididymis.

fluid in the scrotal sac is readily detected as an anechoic band surrounding the testicle. There may be echoes within the fluid depending on its nature (e.g. pus, clotting blood). In epididymitis, enlargement of the epididymis may be detected (Fig. 4.11). In addition, a collection of small cysts may be found adjacent to the testicle, representing fluid distension of the spermatic cord. A similar ultrasonographic appearance may be seen because of a varicocoele (dilated veins arising from the pampiniform plexus).

The presence of abdominal viscera in the scrotal sac, resulting from a scrotal hernia is usually readily detected clinically. In cases of doubt, the presence of tissue adjacent to or surrounding the normal testicle can be confirmed. If bowel loops are present, there will be a heterogenous appearance and acoustic shadowing is likely due to intraluminal gas. If only omental fat is present, irregular echogenic masses will be seen.

Further reading

Bondestam, S., Alitalo, I. and Karkkainen, M. (1983) Real time ultrasound pregnancy diagnosis in the bitch. *Journal of Small Animal Practice*, **24**, 145–151.

Cartee, R.E. and Rowles, T. (1984) Preliminary study of the ultrasonographic diagnosis of pregnancy and foetal development in the dog. *American Journal of Veterinary Research*, **45**, 1259–1265.

Davidson, A.P., Nyland, T.G. and Tsutsui, T. (1986) Pregnancy diagnosis with ultrasound in the domestic cat. *Veterinary Radiology*, **27**, 109–114.

England, G.C.W. and Allen, W.E. (1989) Ultrasonographic and histological appearance of the canine ovary. *Veterinary Record*, **125**, 555–556.

Holst, P.A. and Phemister, R.D. (1974) Onset of diestrus in the beagle bitch: definition and significance. *American Journal of Veterinary Research*, **35**, 401–406.

Inaba, T., Matsui, N., Shimizu, R. and Imori, T. (1984) Use of echography in bitches for detection of ovulation and pregnancy. *Veterinary Record*, **115**, 276–277.

Johnston, S.D., Smith, F.O., Bailie, N.C., Johnston, G.R. and Feeney, D.A. (1983) Prenatal indicators of puppy viability at term. *Compendium of Continuing Education*, **5**, 1013–1024.

Poffenbarger, E.M. and Feeney, D.A. (1986) Use of gray-scale ultrasonography in the diagnosis of reproductive disease in the bitch: 18 cases. *Journal of the American Veterinary Medical Association*, **189**, 90–95.

Shille, M. and Gontarek, J. (1985) The use of ultrasonography for pregnancy diagnosis in the bitch. *Journal of the American Veterinary Medical Association*, **187**, 1021–1025.

Toal, R.L., Walker, M.A. and Henry, G.A. (1986) A comparison of real time ultrasound, palpation and radiography in pregnancy detection and litter size determination in the bitch. *Veterinary Radiology*, **27**, 102–108.

5/Imaging of other Abdominal Structures

The abdominal cavity

Imaging procedure

The abdominal cavity may be examined from any part of the abdominal wall as long as gas-filled viscera and skeletal structures are avoided. The positioning of the animal is therefore not critical and can be chosen to ensure that it is comfortable and relaxed.

If a palpable abdominal mass is present, clearly the sound beam should be directed towards the mass. In cases where there is no palpable abnormality, a systematic search of the abdominal cavity should be made, identifying and examining the major organs as described in the preceding chapters. If free abdominal fluid is suspected, a careful examination of the dependent portions of the abdomen should always be made.

Normal appearance

The abdominal wall itself is rarely defined unless a very close focussing transducer is used. The most superficial tissue which may be identified is intra-abdominal fat, particularly in the regions of the falciform ligament and the ventral ligament of the bladder. The presence of significant amounts of intra-abdominal fat is variable, depending largely on bodily condition. Fat in the ventral midline appears as a smooth, undulating, hypoechoic mass adherent to the abdominal wall. In the normal abdomen this fat is easily overlooked, but in the presence of ascites it is highlighted and may become very obvious. It should be recognized as a normal feature.

In the sublumbar region, the sublumbar muscles can usually be identified ventral to the bodies of the lumbar vertebrae. They are usually hypoechoic and with high resolution images a linear pattern depicting the orientation of the muscle fibres may be recognized. Ventral to the sublumbar muscles in the midline the major abdominal blood vessels can usually be identified. The caudal vena cava is a broad, well-defined, anechoic tubular structure which runs along the length of the abdomen and passes through the diaphragm. The vessel walls are not usually obvious. Pulsations may be noted due to referred movement from the adjacent aorta. The major veins joining the caudal vena cava may also be recognized (e.g. renal veins, hepatic veins). The aorta runs adjacent to the caudal vena cava, but its thicker walls and relatively small lumen make it more difficult to identify. In the cranial abdomen the portal vein may also be seen, lying ventral to the aorta and caudal vena cava.

Normal intra-abdominal lymph nodes are not visible ultrasonographically.

Abnormalities of the abdominal cavity

Free abdominal fluid is readily detected ultrasonographically. Small quantities of free fluid may be found separating the liver lobes, between the liver and the diaphragm, and lying in the dependent portions of the abdomen. These small collections of free fluid tend to be angular in outline and indented by adjacent structures, and they will move when the position of the animal is changed. Large quantities of fluid outline and separate the abdominal viscera (Fig. 5.1).

Abdominal fluid in dogs and cats tends to be anechoic irrespective of its nature (blood, urine, transudate, exudate). Pus may contain some echoes depending on its consistency, so the identification of free abdominal fluid containing swirling particles is suggestive of severe peritonitis. If multiple echogenic strands are visible in the fluid, if the bowel loops are matted together, or if the fluid is loculated, an exudative or neoplastic process is likely. Such features are rarely seen when a transudate is present.

The ultrasonographic detection of free air in the abdomen in man has been reported. Air interferes with image quality and will rise to the uppermost part of the abdomen. Consistent image interference in the uppermost part of the abdomen which shifts as the patient changes position is said to be characteristic of free air. However radiography is probably a more sensitive method of detecting pneumoperitoneum.

Abdominal masses which do not arise from any of the major organs may be detected ultrasonographically depending on their size and position. The echogenicity and architecture of these masses are variable and it is not usually possible to

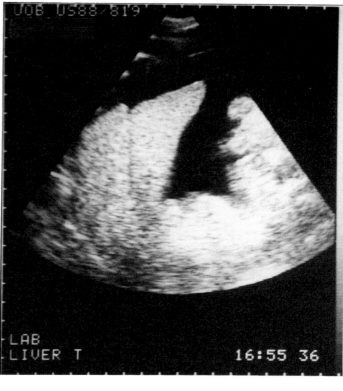

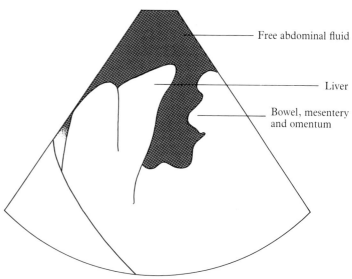

Free abdominal fluid

Liver

Bowel, mesentery and omentum

Fig. 5.1 Ascites in a Labrador. Free abdominal fluid outlines and separates the lobes of the liver and bowel–mesentery–omentum.

determine the histological type from the ultrasonographic appearance. Multicentric lymphosarcoma may cause enlargement of clusters of intra-abdominal lymph nodes. These lymph nodes are seen as rounded, well-circumscribed masses which are evenly hypoechoic (Fig. 5.2), but the appearance is

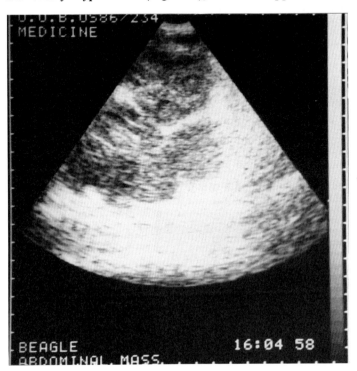

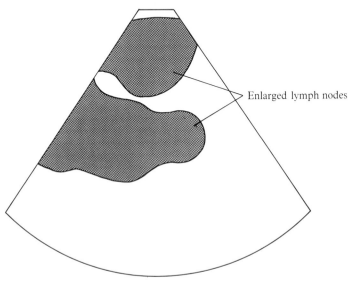

Enlarged lymph nodes

Fig. 5.2 Multicentric lymphosarcoma in a Beagle. The lobulated hypoechoic masses represent enlarged mesenteric lymph nodes.

nonspecific and may also be seen when lymph nodes enlarge due to inflammatory processes. When neoplasms other than lymphosarcoma involve the lymph nodes, abdominal masses of variable ultrasonographic appearance are seen (Fig. 5.3).

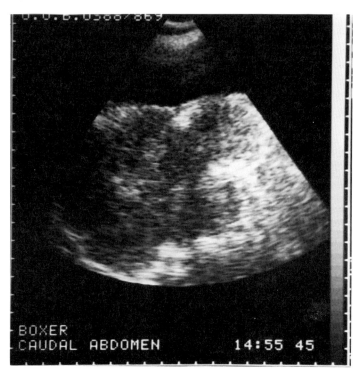

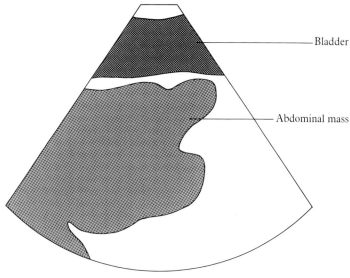

Bladder

Abdominal mass

Fig. 5.3 Abdominal sarcoma in a Boxer. A large, lobulated, hypoechoic mass is situated in the caudal abdomen, dorsal to the bladder.

Although the majority of abdominal masses in the dog and cat are neoplastic, abscesses, cysts and haematomata may also occur. The ultrasonographic criteria for the diagnosis of a simple cyst have already been described — a thin, well-defined wall, anechoic contents and distal acoustic enhancement. Abscesses and haematomata have a variable ultrasonographic appearance but are usually of mixed echogenicity. An abscess may contain gas which is due to gas-forming organisms. Small bubbles will appear ultrasonographically as strongly echogenic particles (Fig. 5.4). If the accumulations of gas are large enough, strong acoustic shadows should be cast. A simple haematoma should slowly resolve and this will be detected on sequential ultrasonographic examinations. However, it may prove impossible to differentiate a tumour with a necrotic centre from an abscess or a haematoma using ultrasonographic criteria alone.

The adrenal glands

Imaging procedure

The normal adrenal glands lie medial and slightly cranial to the cranial pole of each kidney. Therefore, the technique for ultrasonographic examination of the kidneys may be used when searching for the adrenal glands.

The flanks should be clipped just below the sublumbar muscles behind the last rib on the left and over the last two intercostal spaces on the right. With the transducer placed perpendicular to the skin of the prepared area and the plane of the beam parallel to the lumbar spine, the ipsilateral kidney will be seen in coronal section. The caudal vena cava can be identified in longitudinal section medial to the kidney, although it may be necessary to angle the beam slightly dorsally to locate the vessel. The area between the cranial pole of the kidney and the caudal vena cava should be searched meticulously for the adrenal gland. The procedure should then be repeated on the other side.

When searching for the left adrenal gland it is important to realize that part of the spleen and the transverse and descending colon may lie near the cranial pole of the left kidney and mimic an adrenal mass. It should be possible to confirm the identity of both colon and spleen by imaging in more than one plane of section.

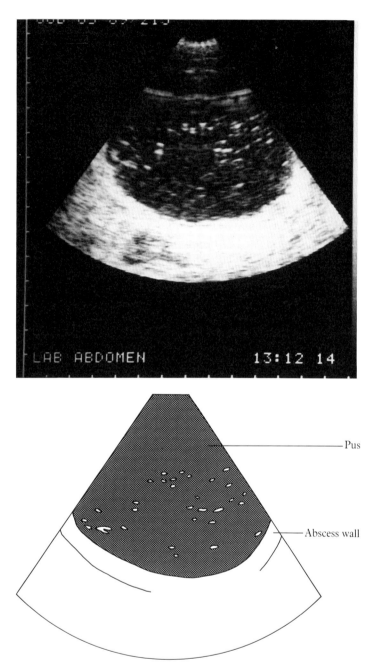

Fig. 5.4 Abdominal abscess in a Labrador. The echogenic particles within the fluid represent gas bubbles.

Normal appearance

The ultrasonographic appearance of normal adrenal glands in the dog has been described. Small flattened triangular masses of moderate echogenicity lie cranial and/or medial to the cranial pole of each kidney. However, the normal adrenal glands are difficult to detect in the dog and cat and are usually not recognized. This is partly because the glands are small and partly because they are often embedded in perirenal fat.

Abnormalities of the adrenal glands

Hyperadrenocorticism in the dog (Cushing's syndrome) is usually associated with some degree of adrenal enlargement. This may take the form of pituitary-dependent adrenal hyperplasia or primary adrenal neoplasia.

An enlarged adrenal gland may be detected ultrasonographically if it is big enough. In the literature, the smallest adrenal mass imaged to date in the dog was 1.4 cm in diameter. However, even large masses may be missed because of overlying bowel or perirenal fat. Most masses are ovoid or spherical in shape and of similar echogenicity to the renal cortex (Fig. 5.5). Strongly echogenic patches with acoustic shadowing indicate mineralization within the mass. In the dog this is suggestive of adrenal neoplasia rather than hyperplasia.

It is important to make a meticulous search for the adrenal glands on both sides. Detection of a unilateral mass suggests a diagnosis of adrenal neoplasia rather than hyperplasia, although the possibility of failing to locate the second hyperplastic gland must be borne in mind. Detection of bilateral adrenal masses indicates pituitary-dependent hyperplasia, although bilateral adrenal tumours have been reported.

Adrenal masses that are not associated with hyperadrenocorticism may also occur. Most adrenocortical tumours are non-functional and any clinical signs which occur may be due to local invasion or compression or due to metastatic disease. Occasionally tumours of the adrenal medulla occur. The histological type of such masses cannot be ascertained from the ultrasonographic appearance.

In the cat, adrenal masses (whether hyperplastic or neoplastic) are less common. It should be recognized that calcification within the adrenal glands in the older cat may be a normal finding.

If an adrenal mass is detected in the dog or cat, it is important to examine the caudal vena cava carefully (Fig. 5.6). If the mass envelops the vena cava or invades the lumen, the likelihood of surgical success is diminished and the overall prognosis is worse.

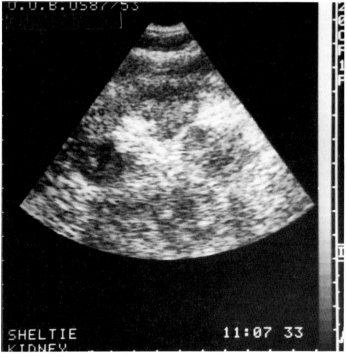

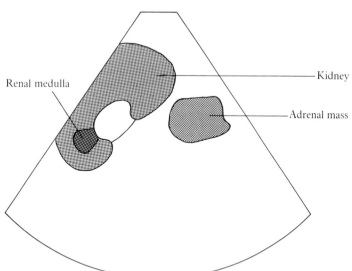

Renal medulla

Kidney

Adrenal mass

Fig. 5.5 Adrenal adenoma in a Shetland Sheepdog. An irregular, hypoechoic mass is located medial to the cranial pole of one kidney.

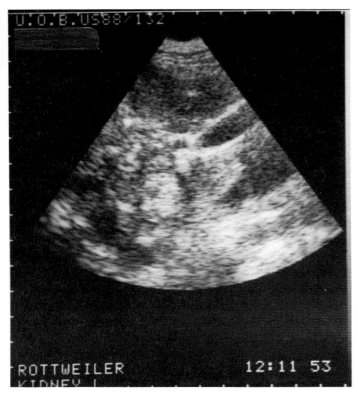

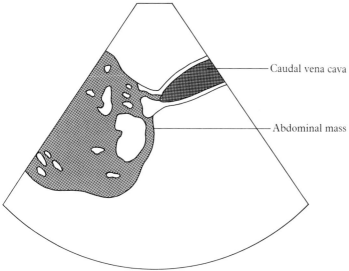

Caudal vena cava

Abdominal mass

Fig. 5.6 Local extension of a renal tumour in a Rottweiler. A poorly defined, heterogeneous mass encircles and compresses the caudal vena cava.

The pancreas

Imaging procedure

The canine pancreas is difficult to examine ultrasonographically. It consists of two long branches — the right branch lies dorsal to the descending duodenum and ventral to the right kidney and the caudate lobe of the liver, while the left branch runs between the gastric antrum and the transverse colon, dorsal to the spleen. The close anatomical relationship of the pancreas to the stomach and duodenum means that gastrointestinal gas often obscures the pancreas completely.

It is vital that the patient is starved prior to ultrasonographic examination of the pancreas, as a stomach containing food will certainly prevent visualization of the pancreas. It can be useful to allow the animal to drink prior to the examination as a fluid-filled stomach and duodenum act as useful landmarks. This may be contraindicated however if acute pancreatitis is suspected, as the ingestion of fluid is likely to induce pancreatic secretion and further vomiting. The animal should be placed in dorsal recumbency and the entire ventral abdomen between the xiphisternum and the umbilicus should be clipped. It is important to extend the clipped area generously on each side of the midline. After routine skin preparation, a search for the pancreas may begin.

Place the transducer to the left of the midline, just behind the costal arch, and angle the sound beam craniodorsally. The gastric fundus should then be visible. If the stomach contains fluid, the outline is well-defined and it is possible to move the transducer to the right to the antrum and pylorus, and then to turn caudally to follow the descending duodenum. Using these landmarks the region of the pancreas can be identified.

More often, the stomach and/or duodenum contain significant amounts of gas, which results in acoustic shadowing. This can make it difficult to follow the path above. In such cases the right kidney should be located by placing the transducer to the right of the midline, just behind the costal arch. It may be necessary to apply gentle but firm downward pressure to displace gas-filled bowel from the area. The right branch of the pancreas should lie ventral to the right kidney. In the midline, the aorta, caudal vena cava and portal vein may all be identified and used as extra landmarks.

It may prove impossible to image the region of the pancreas with the animal in dorsal recumbency because of interference by gastrointestinal gas. Two manoeuvres have been suggested to overcome this. The animal may be placed in right lateral recumbency so that gas in the stomach and bowel rises to the left. The transducer can then be held close to the table to image the right cranioventral abdomen as described above. Alternatively, the animal may be placed in left lateral recumbency and the right kidney located from a right intercostal approach. The pancreatic region should be ventral to the right kidney.

It has been suggested that sterile saline should be instilled into the abdomen to outline the viscera and facilitate ultrasonographic examination of the pancreas. Although the pancreas is then easier to recognize, the disadvantages of the procedure must also be considered before deciding to adopt this method. The abdominal distension may be uncomfortable for the animal, and there is the risk of introducing or disseminating infection in the abdominal cavity.

The indications for ultrasonographic examination of the pancreas in the cat are fewer than in the dog, but the imaging procedure is the same.

Normal appearance

The normal pancreas in the dog and cat is difficult to recognize ultrasonographically. This is partly due to the technical imaging problems discussed above. However, the normal pancreas is also a slender organ with rather poorly defined boundaries, and it is usually surrounded by fat. The region of the pancreas can be identified using the landmarks described above. This area is usually hyperechoic relative to the renal cortex and liver. However, in the normal dog and cat the pancreas is not visible as a discrete organ.

Abnormalities of the pancreas

Acute pancreatitis may be difficult to diagnose in the dog as the clinical signs, although often severe, are non-specific. The characteristic laboratory and radiographic findings are not always present. There have been two published reports to date of the ultrasonographic appearance of experimentally induced pancreatitis in the dog. The most consistent finding was the presence of heterogeneous but predominantly hypoechoic masses in the region of the pancreas. Subsequent post mortem examination showed that these masses represent areas of oedema, inflammation and haemorrhage. Small amounts of free abdominal fluid were often detected in the early stages. In addition, the descending loop of the duodenum often appeared dilated, fluid-filled and hypomotile with a thickened wall. Although the ultrasonographic changes may be less dramatic in the naturally occurring disease, it seems likely that ultrasound can make a useful contribution towards the diagnosis of acute pancreatitis in the dog.

There have been no published reports of the ultrasonographic appearance of pancreatic disorders in the cat. Traumatic pancreatitis in the cat is not common, but may occur as a sequel to road traffic accidents, falling from a height or penetrating wounds. It is likely that the ultrasonographic features of traumatic pancreatitis would resemble those described above for acute pancreatitis.

In chronic pancreatitis, similar masses may be detected in the region of the pancreas. These masses may contain hyperechoic patches representing areas of fibrosis or calcification, or may appear indistinguishable from those associated with acute pancreatitis. The history and clinical signs should usually allow differentiation of acute and chronic pancreatitis.

Pancreatic tumours may be detected ultrasonographically if they are large enough. Insulinomata are often small and so are frequently missed even during a meticulous examination. Exocrine pancreatic tumours usually present at a fairly advanced stage. In such cases a large mass in the region of the pancreas may be detected. The ultrasonographic appearance is variable and it may not be possible to differentiate a pancreatic neoplasm and chronic pancreatitis using ultrasonographic criteria alone. It is important to search for evidence of metastatic disease in the liver. In the absence of metastases, a biopsy may be required to allow a definitive diagnosis.

Enlargement of the pancreas for any reason may result in obstruction of the bile duct and subsequent development of jaundice. The characteristic ultrasonographic features of obstructive jaundice may then be seen on examination of the liver.

The gastrointestinal tract

Imaging procedure

The gastrointestinal tract does not, in general, lend itself to ultrasonographic examination. The presence of solid ingesta or faecal material, and in particular the accumulation of intraluminal gas, impairs image quality. It is also difficult to localize any abnormality found to a specific region of bowel. The advent of endoscopic ultrasound has largely overcome these problems. A high resolution, close focussing transducer with a 360° field of view is mounted on a flexible endoscope and introduced into the appropriate part of the gastrointestinal tract. The transducer can thus be placed in direct contact with the mucosal surface and a high-quality image of the tract wall produced. However, endoscopic ultrasound requires specialized equipment and is still not widely available.

It is possible nevertheless to gain a limited amount of information from conventional ultrasonographic examination of the gastrointestinal tract. In order to investigate the stomach and duodenum, the animal should be starved but allowed to drink prior to the examination. This should ensure that the stomach and duodenum are fluid-filled and therefore clearly delineated. The animal should be placed in dorsal recumbency and the entire ventral abdomen clipped. After routine skin preparation, the transducer should be placed behind the costal arch to the left of the midline and the sound beam angled craniodorsally. Once the gastric fundus has been identified, the transducer can be moved to the right to image the antrum and pylorus, and then caudally to follow the duodenum. The rest of the small intestine can be imaged from the mid-ventral abdominal wall, although the presence of intra-luminal gas often renders the examination unrewarding. The large intestine often contains faecal material so it may be necessary to administer an enema. It is then possible to infuse warm water or saline into the colon and image the resulting fluid-filled structure ultrasonographically. This is not usually practicable as the procedure is poorly tolerated by the conscious animal.

The role of conventional ultrasound in examination of the gastrointestinal tract is limited, and plain and contrast radiography will almost invariably provide more useful information. Nevertheless, the gastrointestinal tract should not be ignored when performing ultrasonographic examinations of the abdomen. It is worth remembering that barium sulphate interferes with image quality so that ultrasonography should precede contrast radiography if barium is to be used. Water soluble iodinated contrast media do not cause the same problems.

Normal appearance

The fluid-filled stomach is a well-circumscribed, pear-shaped structure with a thin, well-defined wall. Since the contents are fluid they appear anechoic, but there are often multiple echogenic particles within the fluid representing small air bubbles (Fig. 5.7). Peristaltic activity may be apparent. The pylorus is often seen as an oval or round distinct mass to the right of the midline and caudal to the liver. It is usually of mixed echogenicity.

The small intestine is only clearly seen if it is fluid-filled. Narrow anechoic tubular structures may be seen in longitudinal or transverse section. The most certain way to differentiate fluid-filled bowel from blood vessels or fluid-filled uterus is to watch for peristalsis.

The detail of the stomach or intestinal wall which is seen depends partly on image quality but mostly on the resolving power of the transducer selected. With most standard abdominal frequencies (3.5–7.5 MHz) the wall appears as a uniform hypoechoic structure. There may be a central echogenic core representing the interface between the mucosa and the lumen. If a high-resolution transducer (10 MHz) is available, five distinct layers may be recognized (Fig. 5.8).

1 Hyperechoic inner layer — interface between mucosa and lumen.
2 Hypoechoic layer — mucosa.
3 Hyperechoic middle layer — submucosa.
4 Hypoechoic layer — muscle.
5 Hyperechoic outer layer — boundary between the serosa and the peritoneal cavity.

Abnormalities of the gastrointestinal tract

Only gross abnormalities of the gastrointestinal tract will be recognized using conventional ultrasonographic techniques.

Abnormal fluid distension of the stomach may be seen in cases of pyloric outflow obstruction, although the assessment of gastric size remains subjective at present. It is sometimes possible to appreciate vigorous peristaltic contractions without effective gastric emptying. Gaseous distension of the stomach, as occurs in acute gastric dilation/torsion, cannot be properly assessed ultrasonographically.

Distension of loops of small intestine associated with paralytic ileus or mechanical obstruction may be seen if the loops

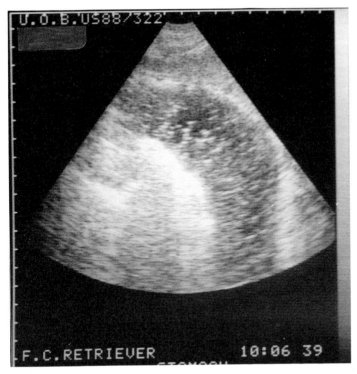

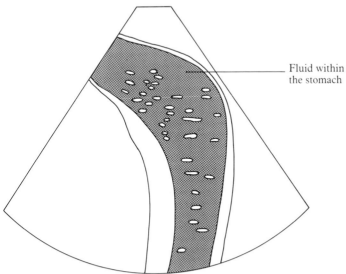

Fluid within
the stomach

Fig. 5.7 Normal stomach in a
Flat Coat Retriever. The wall
of the stomach is not clearly
defined, but the fluid contents
are visible. Echogenic particles
within the fluid represent gas
bubbles and/or food particles.

are fluid-filled. Once again, gaseous distension precludes accurate evaluation of the small intestine.

Mucosal abnormalities and small changes in thickness of
the bowel wall are not detected by conventional ultrasound.

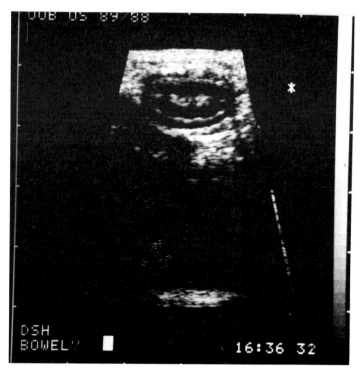

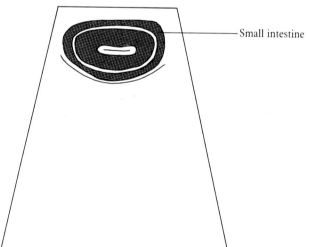

Small intestine

Fig. 5.8 Normal small intestine in a cat. This high-resolution image shows a transverse section through small intestine. The classical five layers can be recognized.

However, gross bowel wall thickening may be recognized. The ultrasonographic appearance of abdominal masses which are intestinal in origin is quite typical (Fig. 5.9). They tend to be rounded, quite well circumscribed and hypoechoic. The centre of the mass is typically echogenic due to the acoustic interface between the mucosal surface and the lumen. Some-

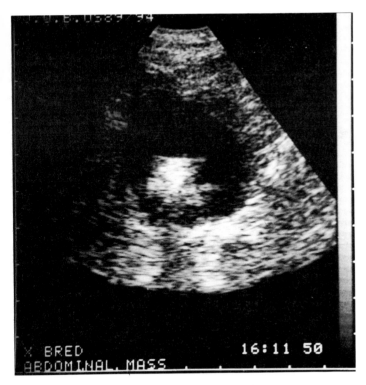

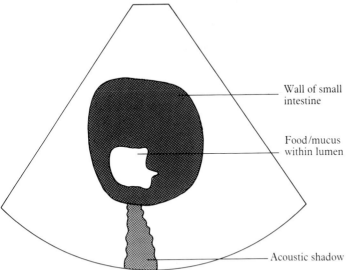

Wall of small intestine

Food/mucus within lumen

Acoustic shadow

Fig. 5.9 Tumour of the small intestine in a cross-breed dog. The eccentric thickening of the intestinal wall around the lumen is suggestive of neoplasia. The acoustic shadow may be due to gas or mineral fragments within the lumen.

times acoustic shadows are seen, owing to the trapping of particulate mineralized material in the lumen.

It should be emphasized that ultrasound at present remains of limited use in evaluation of the gastrointestinal tract.

Further reading

Feeney, D.A., Johnston, G.R. and Walter, P.A. (1985) Two-dimensional gray-scale abdominal ultrasonography: general interpretation and abdominal masses. *Veterinary Clinics of North America: Small Animal Practice*, **15**, 1225–1248.

Kantrowitz, B.M., Nyland, T.G. and Feldman, E.C. (1986) Adrenal ultrasonography in the dog. *Veterinary Radiology*, **27**, 91–96.

Kantrowitz, B.M., Dimski, D., Swalec, K. and Biller, D.S. (1988) Ultrasonographic detection of jejunal intussusception and acute renal failure due to ethylene glycol toxicity in a dog. *Journal of the American Animal Hospital Association*, **24**, 697–700.

Konde, L.J., Lebel, J.L., Park, R.D. and Wrigley, R.H. (1986) Sonographic application in the diagnosis of intra-abdominal abscess in the dog. *Veterinary Radiology*, **27**, 151–154.

Miles, K.G., Lattimer, J.C., Krause, G.F., Knapp, D.W. and Sayles, C.E. (1988) The use of intraperitoneal fluid as a simple technique for enhancing sonographic visualisation of the canine pancreas. *Veterinary Radiology*, **29**, 258–263.

Murtaugh, R.J., Herring, D.S., Jacobs, R.M. and DeHoff, W.D. (1985) Pancreatic ultrasonography in dogs with experimentally induced acute pancreatitis. *Veterinary Radiology*, **26**, 27–32.

Nyland, T.G., Mulvaney, M.H. and Strombeck, D.R. (1983) Ultrasonic features of experimentally induced acute pancreatitis in the dog. *Veterinary Radiology*, **24**, 260–266.

Poffenbarger, E.M., Feeney, D.A. and Hayden, D.W. (1988) Gray-scale ultrasonography in the diagnosis of adrenal neoplasia in dogs: six cases (1981–1986). *Journal of the American Veterinary Medical Association*, **192**, 228–232.

6/Imaging of the Heart — Echocardiography

Imaging procedure

The selection of an appropriate acoustic window is particularly critical when imaging the heart. Bone and gas will block the passage of ultrasound, so it is necessary to choose a scanning area which avoids the skeletal structures of the thoracic wall and where there is minimal air-filled lung interposed between the transducer and the heart. This is achieved by placing the transducer between the ribs low down on the thoracic wall. In order to perform a thorough cardiac evaluation, the heart should be imaged from both the left and right. A small area of hair should be clipped extending for several intercostal spaces over the palpable apex beat on each side of the thorax (usually between ribs four and six). Routine skin preparation should then be carried out.

It is helpful to have a working surface with a small hole cut from it. This allows the animal to be placed on its side and the heart imaged from beneath, minimizing interference from air-filled lung. When the heart has been imaged from one side, the animal can be turned over and the procedure repeated from the other side. If this is not possible the heart may be imaged from above (Fig. 6.1), although interference from air-filled lung may then be a problem, particularly in barrel-chested dogs. If the animal becomes distressed when restrained on its side, the heart can be imaged with the patient standing or sitting. The front leg should be pulled forward gently to facilitate access to the appropriate part of the thoracic wall.

Sedation and general anaesthesia should be avoided where possible during ultrasonographic evaluation of the heart since cardiac rate, rhythm and contractility may be altered.

The equipment used is of particular importance in cardiac ultrasonography. A transducer with a small contact surface is essential to allow access between the ribs. A sector scanner is necessary to enable flexibility in imaging planes. A 3.5 or 5 MHz transducer is quite adequate for the examination of the heart of large- and medium-sized dogs. In small dogs and cats

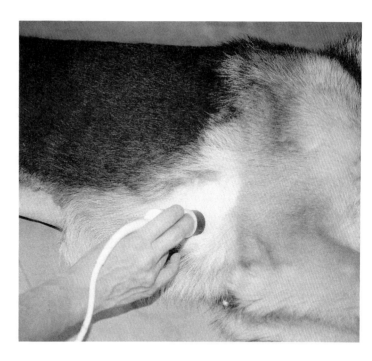

Fig. 6.1 Imaging the heart from the right thoracic wall.

a 7.5 MHz transducer with close focussing may be necessary in order to achieve resolution of anatomical structures.

It is important to establish a protocol for ultrasonographic examination of the heart to ensure that nothing is missed. By altering the plane of section of the beam, the chambers, valves and great vessels can all be identified from the real-time two-dimensional images, and subjective assessments made of cardiac and valvular motility. Cardiac dimensions can be measured on frozen two-dimensional images provided care is taken to standardize the plane of section and the stage of the cardiac cycle is noted using a simultaneous ECG recording. However, accurate quantitative analysis is probably better performed on standard M mode traces. The required plane of section should be imaged using the two-dimensional display mode. The M mode cursor may then be carefully positioned across the structures of interest before selecting the M mode display. The measurements made can be related to body weight or surface area and compared with the published normal values for the dog and cat.

It is worth stressing that a meticulous cardiac examination takes time, and if attempts are made to hurry or miss out steps then valuable information may be missed. It is useful to record each examination on videotape as this allows subsequent re-evaluation of the images, if necessary frame-by-frame. This is particularly important in small dogs and cats where the heart rate may be very fast.

Normal appearance

The aim of the cardiac examination is to: (i) identify the four chambers of the heart and their relationship with each other; (ii) note the cardiac rate and rhythm; (iii) evaluate the motion of the ventricular walls and the interventricular septum; (iv) assess the internal systolic and diastolic dimensions and the wall thickness of each chamber; (v) look for masses within each chamber or involving the myocardium; (vi) examine the integrity of the interatrial and interventricular septum; (vii) look at the atrioventricular valves, chordae tendineae and papillary muscles, considering both structure and function; (viii) locate the right and left ventricular outflow tracts and evaluate outflow diameter and valvular structure and function; and (ix) assess the thickness of the epicardium/pericardium and search for evidence of fluid or masses within the pericardial space. It is also important to search for evidence of cardiac failure (e.g. pleural fluid, hepatic venous congestion, ascites).

One possible protocol for ultrasonographic examination of the heart is shown below. It is important to realize that the precise orientation of the heart may vary with breed conformation and intrathoracic pathology.

From the right

1. Short axis views ('Transverse sections')

Begin with the plane of the beam parallel to the sternum, then adjust the angle until an accurate short-axis view is seen. This shows the left ventricle as a circular structure with the right ventricle wrapped around it. Start near the apex of the heart and angle progressively up towards the base (Figs 6.2, 6.3, 6.4).

2. Long axis views ('Longitudinal sections')

Rotate the transducer through approximately 90° from the short axis view, then make fine adjustments as necessary in

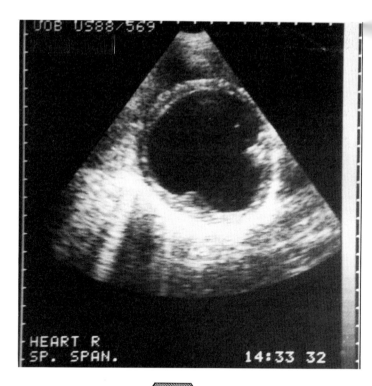

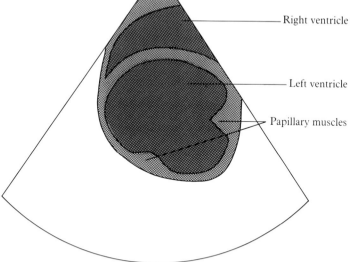

Right ventricle

Left ventricle

Papillary muscles

Fig. 6.2 Short axis view of the heart at the level of the papillary muscles, imaged from the right thoracic wall, in a Springer Spaniel. This heart is not normal — the left ventricle is dilated.

order to identify the following planes of section. The plane of the beam should be rotated a few degrees clockwise in order to move from view **a** to view **b**:

a View optimized for the left atrium and mitral valve (Fig. 6.5).

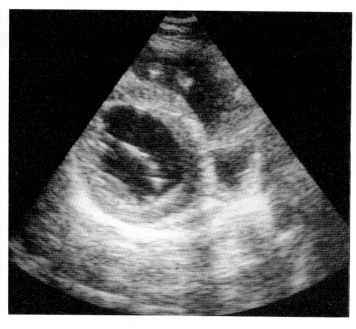

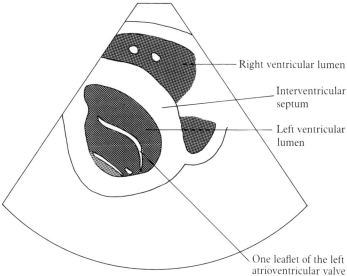

Right ventricular lumen

Interventricular septum

Left ventricular lumen

One leaflet of the left atrioventricular valve

Fig. 6.3 Short axis view of the normal heart at the level of the atrioventricular valves, imaged from the right thoracic wall in a Greyhound. The left atrioventricular valve is seen *en face*.

b View optimized for the left ventricular outflow tract and aortic valve (Fig. 6.6).
c View between these two showing parts of both the outflow tract and the left atrium.

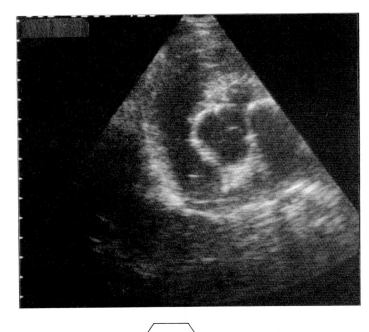

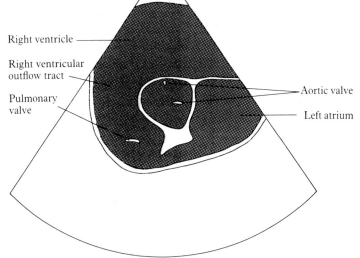

Right ventricle

Right ventricular
outflow tract

Pulmonary
valve

Aortic valve

Left atrium

Fig. 6.4 Short axis view of
the normal heart at the level of
the heart base, imaged from the
right thoracic wall, in a
Lurcher. The aortic valve is
seen *en face* and has a typical
clover-leaf appearance. The
right ventricular outflow tract
and pulmonary valve are seen
in longitudinal section.

3. M mode

1 Record in M mode on the short axis view at the level of the
tips of the papillary muscles taking care to place the scan line
between the two papillary muscles (Fig. 6.7).

2 Alternatively, an M mode trace may be recorded on the
long axis view showing both the aortic outflow tract and the

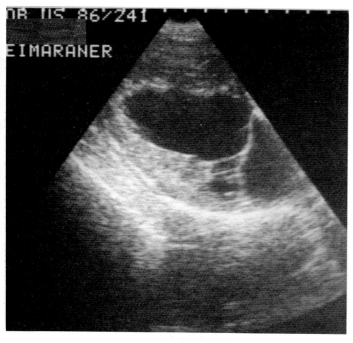

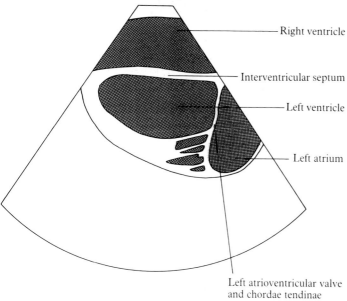

Right ventricle

Interventricular septum

Left ventricle

Left atrium

Left atrioventricular valve
and chordae tendinae

Fig. 6.5 Long axis view of the
normal heart, imaged from the
right thoracic wall, in a
Weimaraner. This view is
angled to show the left atrium,
left ventricle and left
atrioventricular valve.

left atrium. The cursor is placed below the mitral valve but
above the papillary muscle.

Measurements of left ventricular wall thickness and the
internal systolic and diastolic dimensions may be made on

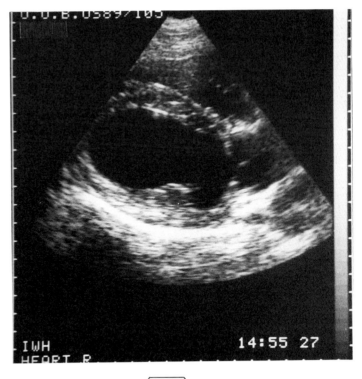

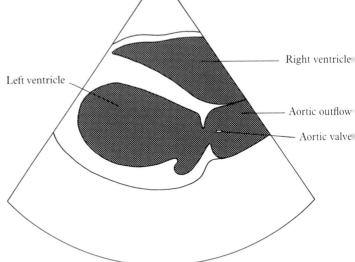

Fig. 6.6 Long axis view of the normal heart, imaged from the right thoracic wall, in an Irish Wolfhound. This view is angled to show the aortic outflow.

either of these images. From the internal systolic (LVs) and diastolic (LVd) dimensions, the ventricular shortening fraction may be calculated ([LVd − LVs] ÷ LVd expressed as a percentage). This gives a measure of myocardial function. Normal

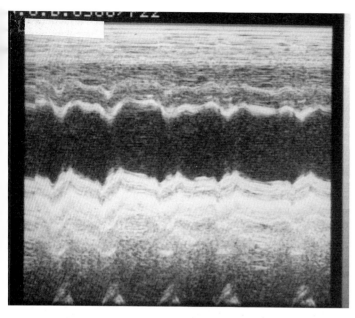

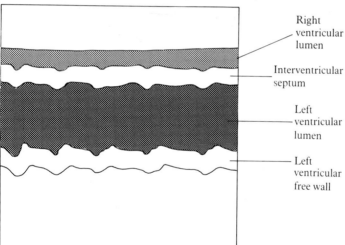

Right ventricular lumen

Interventricular septum

Left ventricular lumen

Left ventricular free wall

Fig. 6.7 Normal M mode in a cross-breed dog, showing motion of the interventricular septum and the left ventricular free wall.

left ventricular shortening fractions have been reported to range from 28–45% in the dog and from 29–55% in the cat.
3 Using the long axis view showing the left ventricular outflow tract and the aortic valve, position the M mode cursor across the aortic root and the left auricle.

The left auricular dimension (LA) and the aortic root diameter (Ao) may be measured, and the ratio LA : Ao measured. This ratio is around 1 : 1 in the normal dog and cat.

In addition, the cursor may be placed across the atrioventricular and aortic valves to allow assessment of the excursion of the valve cusps (Fig. 6.8).

From the left

1. Apical four-chamber view

Place the transducer over the apex beat on the left with the plane of the beam approximately parallel to the sternum, then adjust the plane of the beam until a short-axis view of the heart is achieved. Next, angle the beam steeply upwards along the length of the heart. Fine adjustments should be made to the plane of section until a longitudinal view of all four chambers of the heart is seen (Fig. 6.9).

Contrast techniques

Contrast echocardiography may sometimes be used to confirm or rule out an abnormality suspected from the initial cardiac evaluation. The technique involves the injection of a bolus of contrast agent into the blood-stream while imaging the heart. A cloud of highly echogenic particles can then be seen passing through the chambers of the heart and the great vessels, allowing the pattern of blood flow to be followed and some major anomalies detected (Fig. 6.10). The echoes are caused by microbubbles which may remain stable for 10 s or more but which are usually dissipated in the pulmonary circulation.

Indocyanine green was the first substance discovered to produce echocontrast on intravenous injection. It has since been shown that many fluids, including saline and blood, will produce sparse streams of bubbles if agitated before injection.

A number of 'cocktails' have been investigated in an attempt to increase the contrast achieved and to improve the stability of the microbubbles produced. The introduction of various colloids into these mixtures has certainly improved the quality and stability of the contrast, to the extent that some mixtures are claimed to produce microbubbles which survive the pulmonary circulation. Specialized echocontrast agents are now commercially available.

An effective and widely available echocontrast agent is the colloid 'Haemaccel' (Hoechst Animal Health). A small quantity of this or a similar substance (about 2 ml in a cat, up to 15 ml in a large dog) should be driven back and forth between

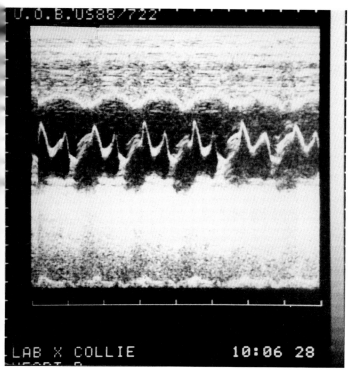

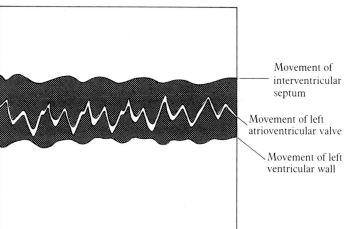

Movement of interventricular septum

Movement of left atrioventricular valve

Movement of left ventricular wall

Fig. 6.8 Normal M mode through the left atrioventricular (mitral) valve in a cross-breed dog. Note the typical 'M' shape traced by the valve.

two syringes through a three-way tap. This provides excellent agitation. The contrast can then be injected as a bolus while the heart is being imaged and the resulting dense echo stream followed.

Non-selective contrast echocardiography entails the injection

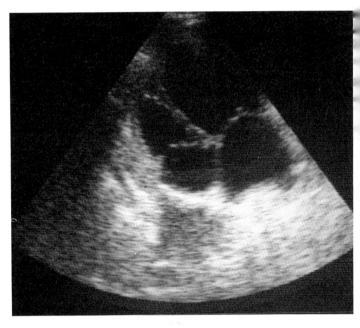

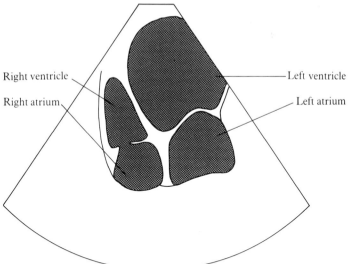

Right ventricle   Left ventricle

Right atrium   Left atrium

Fig. 6.9 Four-chamber view of the heart, imaged from the left thoracic wall, in a Cocker Spaniel. This dog has mild dilation of the left ventricle and left atrium.

of contrast into a peripheral vein. This results in opacification of the right atrium, right ventricle and pulmonary outflow tract, but the microbubbles are usually dissipated in the pulmonary circulation so the left cardiac chambers are not normally opacified. This is a simple, safe and relatively non-invasive procedure which may be performed without general anaesthesia. It has limitations, in that blood flow through the

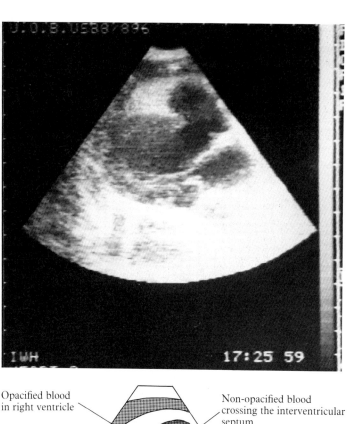

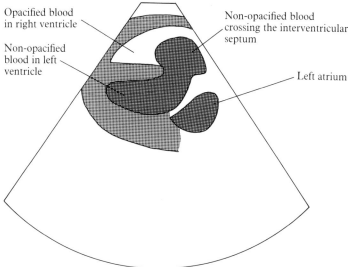

Opacified blood
in right ventricle

Non-opacified blood
crossing the interventricular
septum

Non-opacified
blood in left
ventricle

Left atrium

Fig. 6.10   Ventricular septal
defect in an Irish Wolfhound.
A non-selective echocontrast
technique has been use. Blood
in the right ventricle is
opacified, while blood in the
left atrium and left ventricle is
not opacified. Non-opacified
blood can be seen ballooning
across the interventricular
septum into the right ventricle.

left side of the heart cannot be fully evaluated, and left-to-
right shunting lesions may therefore be difficult to detect.
However, right-to-left shunting lesions may be identified. It is
also possible to perform selective contrast echocardiography

by cardiac catheterization and injection of the contrast at a specific site. Clearly this is a more invasive procedure which requires general anaesthesia, but it may be indicated in some cases.

When performing contrast echocardiography, it is important to avoid injection of large air bubbles as air embolism is a potentially fatal complication. If the solution is well-agitated so that only microbubbles are injected, the procedure is quite safe.

Congenital cardiac disease

Ultrasound is of great value in defining congenital cardiac anomalies in small animals. In many instances the defect may actually be seen. In other cases, the response of the heart to the defect in terms of chamber dilation and/or hypertrophy may be detected and the precise anomaly inferred. Accurate diagnosis of such congenital defects is of importance as this allows appropriate treatment to be instituted in individual animals and an informed prognosis given. It also allows advice to be given on the implications for breeding programmes.

It is important to remember, however, that ultrasound should never be used in isolation, but should rather be considered in conjunction with the history, clinical examination, radiography and electrocardiography.

Patent ductus arteriosus

This is the commonest congenital cardiac anomaly in dogs. It also occurs in cats but far less commonly. In most cases the patent ductus arteriosus itself cannot be recognized. However, the response of the heart to the defect can be seen. The left atrium is moderately dilated owing to the increased volume of blood returning from the lungs. The left ventricle is usually dilated, and mild hypertrophy may also be noted. Ventricular contractility is normal or increased. These changes, with the presence of the characteristic murmur, are sufficient to make a presumptive diagnosis of a patent ductus arteriosus. It is very important to check that there are no other cardiac anomalies as these could affect the prognosis.

Aortic stenosis

Aortic stenosis in the dog is most often subvalvular, although

the valvular type has been reported. In the cat both subvalvular and supravalvular types occur although the latter are said
to be more common.

The most obvious ultrasonographic finding in cases of
moderate−severe aortic stenosis, irrespective of type, is
marked left ventricular hypertrophy. This may be so severe
that the outflow obstruction is exacerbated. There may also
be dilation of the left atrium. Ventricular contractility is normal. In the subvalvular type, a distinct narrowing is often
seen below the aortic valve (Fig. 6.11). This narrowed region
may be noticeably more echogenic than other parts of the
outflow tract, because of a band of fibrous tissue. In the
valvular type, the valve cusps may appear thickened and/or
short, and may seem rather rigid or fixed. In the supravalvular
type, narrowing of the ascending aorta distal to the valve may
be recognized. In all types a marked poststenotic dilation of
the outflow tract may be seen.

Mild aortic stenosis cannot be ruled out by normal two-
dimensional echocardiography. In such cases Doppler techniques are required to demonstrate the abnormal pressure
gradient.

Pulmonary stenosis

Pulmonary stenosis is the second most common congenital
cardiac anomaly in the dog but is rare in the cat. The stenosis
is usually valvular but muscular hypertrophy in the infun-
dibular region of the outflow tract may add to the outflow
obstruction during systole.

The most striking ultrasonographic feature of pulmonary
stenosis is marked right ventricular hypertrophy. In the normal dog and cat the right ventricular wall is approximately
half to one-third the thickness of the left ventricular wall. In
pulmonary stenosis, the thickness of the right ventricular wall
increases until it is equal to, or even exceeds, that of the left
ventricular wall. Abnormal (flat or paradoxical) septal motion
is a finding indicative of right ventricular volume or pressure
overload, and so may be recognized in association with pulmonary stenosis. Paradoxical septal motion is most easily
detected on an M mode trace — the interventricular septum
moves away from, instead of towards, the left ventricular free
wall during systole. Tricuspid insufficiency and right atrial
dilation may also develop as a consequence of the right ventricular dilation.

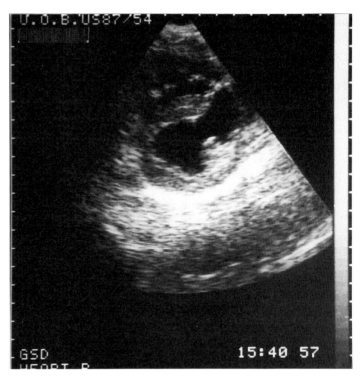

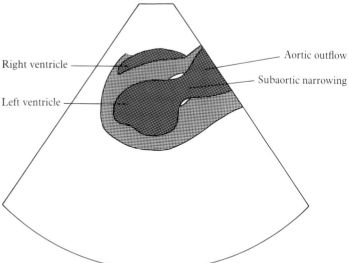

Fig. 6.11 Aortic stenosis in a German Shepherd Dog. A distinct subaortic narrowing and poststenotic dilation can be seen in this long axis view.

The pulmonary outflow tract can be hard to image, but is easiest to find on a short-axis view of the base of the heart from the right thoracic wall. The valve leaflets may look thickened in the valvular form (Fig. 6.12) and there may be

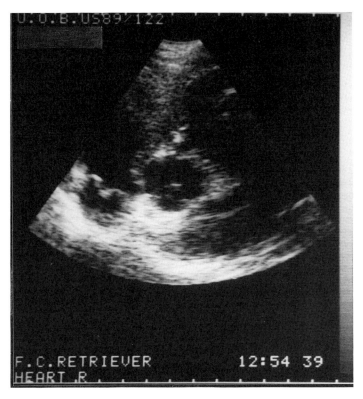

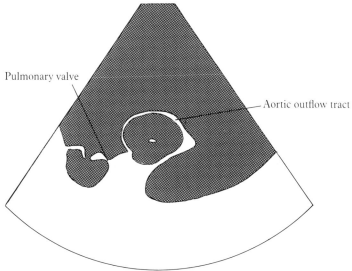

Fig. 6.12 Pulmonary stenosis in a Flat Coat Retriever. This short axis view of the base of the heart shows the thickened, echogenic leaflets of the pulmonary valve.

narrowing of the subvalvular region. A poststenotic dilation may be detected.

It is very important to search the heart for other anomalies, particularly septal defects including those comprising the tetralogy of Fallot. If cyanosis is present, suggesting right-to-left shunting, contrast echocardiography may be indicated.

Atrial septal defect

Atrial septal defects are relatively uncommon. They are classified into two main types. The 'ostium primum' type is an endocardial cushion defect at the atrioventricular junction. This is the more common type in the cat. The 'ostium secundum' type is located in the centre of the interatrial septum, with intact septum above and below the defect (Fig. 6.13). This is the more common type in the dog. Moderately sized and large defects may be seen ultrasonographically if a careful examination of the interatrial septum is made. However, care must be taken as the interatrial septum is a thin structure and 'echo drop-out' in the region of the fossa ovale may simulate a septal defect. Therefore, any defect should ideally be confirmed on more than one view. Contrast echocardiography may be used to confirm a diagnosis of an atrial septal defect. Non-selective techniques normally result in opacification of the right atrium and right ventricle. Under most circumstances, blood will shunt from left to right across an atrial septal defect — thus non-opacified blood may be detected passing across the defect into the opacified blood of the right atrium. Even this finding must be interpreted carefully as the blood in the right atrium is collected from several sources (the cranial vena cava, the caudal vena cava and the coronary sinuses). With cephalic venous injection of contrast, only blood from the cranial vena cava will be opacified.

An atrial septal defect is rarely clinically significant when it occurs in isolation. A large defect may result in volume overload of the right cardiac chambers. Thus, dilation of the right atrium and ventricle, and paradoxical movement of the interventricular septum may be seen ultrasonographically. Atrial septal defects may complicate other cardiac defects.

Ventricular septal defect

Most ventricular septal defects in dogs and cats are located high up in the fibrous part of the interventricular septum, just

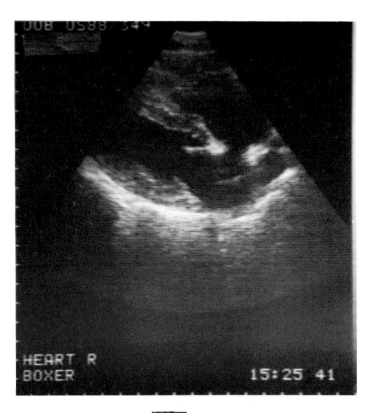

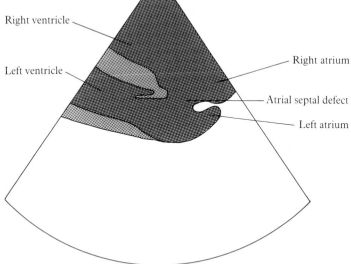

Fig. 6.13 Atrial septal defect in a Boxer. This was an incidental finding.

below the atrioventricular junction. Particularly in cats, such defects may be associated with an 'ostium primum' atrial septal defect, resulting in a common atrioventricular defect. In both dogs and cats, ventricular septal defects may be associated with other congenital anomalies.

If a meticulous search is made of the interventricular septum, the defect itself may be seen. This should be confirmed by identifying the anomaly on more than one plane of section. Once again, contrast echocardiography may be used to confirm doubtful cases. If a non-selective technique is used, a negative jetting effect may be seen as non-opacified blood from the left ventricle crosses the defect to mix with the opacified blood in the right ventricle. If right-to-left shunting is occurring be-cause of increased right ventricular pressure, opacified blood may be seen crossing the defect into the left ventricle. Cardiac catheterization may be used in conjunction with contrast echocardiography if required, but this is rarely necessary.

In the case of left-to-right shunting, volume overload of the right ventricle occurs. Therefore, right ventricular dilation and sometimes hypertrophy may be detected. Dilation of the left atrium may also be seen due to the increased volume of blood returning from the lungs.

Tetralogy of Fallot

This complex cardiac abnormality is found in dogs and cats, but is uncommon. The classical combination of anomalies include pulmonary stenosis and a ventricular septal defect, with varying degrees of dextraposition of the aorta and com-pensatory right ventricular hypertrophy. The most striking ultrasonographic feature is the marked right ventricular hy-pertrophy. In the long axis view from the right, the detection of a high ventricular septal defect differentiates this complex anomaly from an uncomplicated pulmonary stenosis (Fig. 6.14). In classical cases, the aortic outflow can be seen to override the ventricular septum.

Other complex cardiac anomalies may occur and can be difficult to define. The number and relationship of the chambers of the heart, and the connections of the chambers to the great vessels should be determined as far as possible, but selective catheterization and contrast studies may be needed.

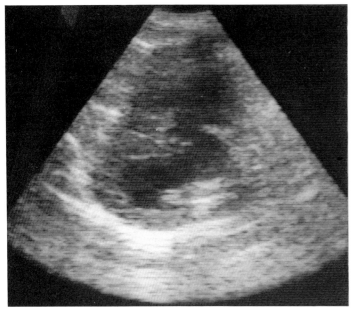

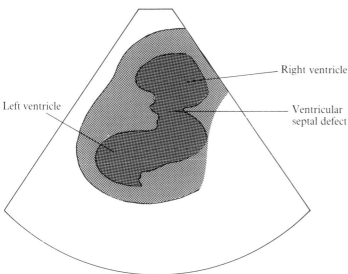

Right ventricle

Left ventricle

Ventricular
septal defect

Fig. 6.14 Tetralogy of Fallot in a Maltese Terrier. This image is of poor quality, but shows a clear ventricular septal defect. There is also dilation and hypertrophy of the right ventricle.

Dysplasia of the atrioventricular valves

Congenital deformities of the left or right atrioventricular valves are seen commonly in cats and occasionally in dogs. They are usually straightforward to identify ultrasonographically. Because of valvular incompetence, extreme dilation of the atrium on the affected side with bowing of the interatrial septum is the most striking feature (Fig. 6.15). The ventricle

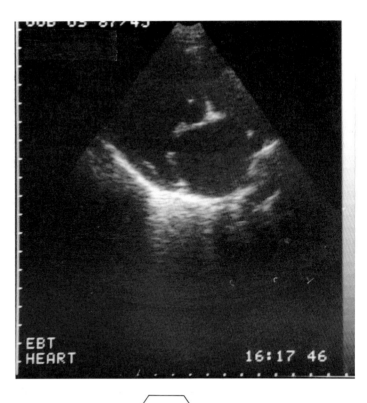

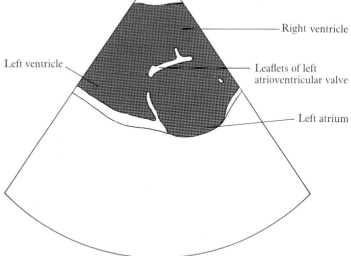

Right ventricle

Left ventricle

Leaflets of left
atrioventricular valve

Left atrium

Fig. 6.15 Dysplasia of the left atrioventricular (mitral) valve in an English Bull Terrier. Note the clubbing of the valve leaflets and the dilation of the left atrium. The interventricular and interatrial septa cannot be clearly distinguished in this image, but were shown to be intact during the rest of the examination.

may show slight hypertrophy, and contractility is likely to be normal or increased unless secondary myocardial failure supervenes. The valve cusps may appear short and thickened, and rather restricted in their movements. This can be aggravated by abnormal development of the chordae tendineae and/or papillary muscles.

Congenital dysplasia of the atrioventricular valves and acquired valvular disease due to endocardiosis or endocarditis may appear similar ultrasonographically, so the age of the animal and the clinical history must be taken into account when reaching a diagnosis.

Acquired cardiac disease

Ultrasonography provides a safe and non-invasive way of diagnosing acquired cardiac disease. Information regarding cardiac function as well as structure is available, thus allowing rational treatment to be employed. Ultrasound lends itself to sequential examinations so the response of the heart to therapy can be monitored.

Insufficiency of the left atrioventricular (mitral) valve

In the small and medium breeds of dog, acquired mitral insufficiency is most commonly due to endocardiosis. The valve leaflets become irregularly thickened and deformed due to progressive non-inflammatory degenerative changes. Acquired mitral insufficiency in the cat and in large and giant breeds of dog usually occurs secondary to cardiomyopathy when the valvular incompetence occurs simply as a result of ventricular dilatation. No structural abnormality of the valve leaflets occurs.

Mitral insufficiency results in dilation of the left atrium, and this is the most prominent feature on ultrasonographic examination (Fig. 6.16). In the absence of myocardial disease, the left ventricle may show varying degrees of dilation and hypertrophy and a normal or increased shortening fraction. These ventricular changes are compensatory changes which help the heart to maintain its output. In the later stages of mitral insufficiency, myocardial disease may supervene so that cardiac motility is decreased.

When mitral insufficiency is due to endocardiosis, the valve leaflets appear irregularly thickened on ultrasonographic examination. It is possible to produce an artefactual appearance of valve thickening by imaging the leaflets obliquely, so it is important to make sure that any changes are consistently visible. Abnormal movement of the leaflets may also be detected. If acute rupture of chordae tendineae occurs, prolapse

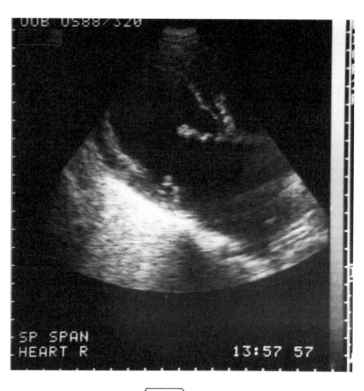

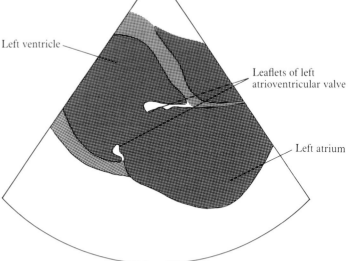

Left ventricle

Leaflets of left
atrioventricular valve

Left atrium

Fig. 6.16 Endocardiosis of
the left atrioventricular (mitral)
valve in a Springer Spaniel.
The valve leaflets are thickened
and irregular. There is marked
dilation of the left atrium and
moderate dilation of the left
ventricle.

of the valve into the left atrium during ventricular systole may
be seen.

Insufficiency of the right atrioventricular (tricuspid) valve

Acquired tricuspid insufficiency in the dog is most commonly
due to endocardiosis and usually occurs in association with
mitral insufficiency. It leads to right atrial dilation, which can
be detected ultrasonographically. The valvular thickenings
associated with endocardiosis may be noted.

Bacterial endocarditis

Bacterial endocarditis is uncommon in dogs and rare in cats.
It most commonly affects the aortic and mitral valves. Ultrasonographically, the valvular vegetations may be detected as
irregularly thickened, echogenic valve leaflets (Fig. 6.17). The
thickenings may be brighter and more irregular than those
seen in endocardiosis, but clearly the history, clinical signs
and results of blood culture must be considered before reaching a definitive diagnosis.

Other ultrasonographic features which may be seen reflect
the results of valvular insufficiency, and will vary according to
the valve(s) involved.

Mild bacterial endocarditis cannot be ruled out by normal
findings on two-dimensional echocardiography.

Cardiomyopathy

Cardiomyopathy may be classified into two main types —
dilated and hypertrophic.

In the dog, idiopathic cardiomyopathy is relatively common
in large and giant breeds but is seen less often than acquired
valvular disease overall. The dilated form occurs more frequently than the hypertrophic form, which is rare. Dilated
cardiomyopathy is readily recognized ultrasonographically.
There is usually moderate–severe left atrial dilation ac-
companied by left ventricular dilation (Fig. 6.18). Right atrial
and ventricular dilation may also be seen, but is usually less
prominent. Myocardial contractility is reduced, resulting in a
low calculated ventricular shortening fraction (Fig. 6.19). The
aortic outflow tract may appear uniformly narrow, reflecting
poor cardiac output. In the hypertrophic form, marked hypertrophy of the ventricular free walls and septum occurs.

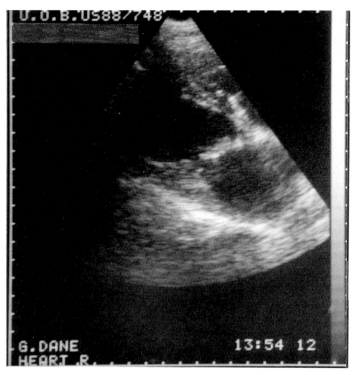

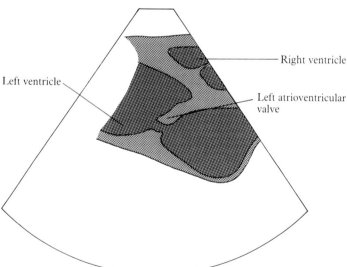

Right ventricle

Left ventricle

Left atrioventricular valve

Fig. 6.17 Endocarditis of the left atrioventricular (mitral) valve in a Great Dane. The valve leaflet is irregularly thickened. This was a consistent finding on more than one plane of section.

The hypertrophy may affect all regions equally or may be asymmetrical in distribution leading to obliteration of the left ventricular outflow tract.

In the cat, cardiomyopathy is by far the commonest form of

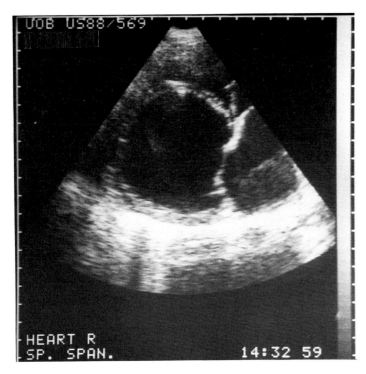

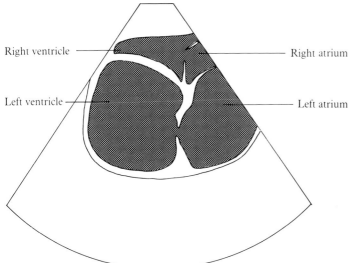

Right ventricle — — Right atrium

Left ventricle — — Left atrium

Fig. 6.18 Dilated cardiomyopathy in a Springer Spaniel. Note the marked dilation of both the left atrium and left ventricle.

acquired heart disease. Both dilated and hypertrophic forms are seen and some cases seem to have features of both forms. Ultrasound allows differentiation of the two types which is of importance when selecting the appropriate treatment. Dilated

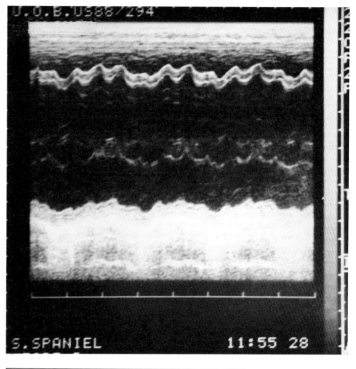

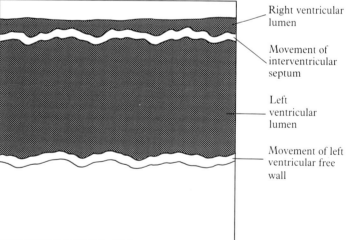

Right ventricular
lumen

Movement of
interventricular
septum

Left
ventricular
lumen

Movement of left
ventricular free
wall

Fig. 6.19 The M mode
tracing of the heart depicted in
Fig. 6.18 shows very poor
myocardial motility.

cardiomyopathy results in the dilation of all four cardiac
chambers. The left ventricular wall has a decreased end-
systolic thickness. Myocardial contractility is clearly diminished. The aortic outflow may be uniformly narrow, because
of the poor cardiac output. Thromboembolism is a common
complication and, in this event, irregular, moderately echoic

masses may be seen in the atria. The characteristic feature of hypertrophic cardiomyopathy is hypertrophy of the ventricular free walls and septum (Fig. 6.20). Biatrial dilation may also be seen. It is important to remember that in the older cat

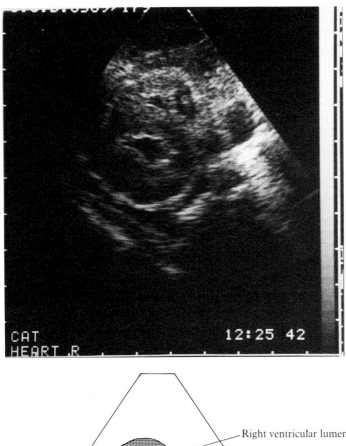

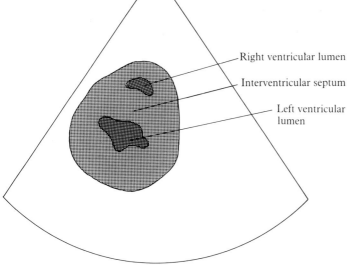

Fig. 6.20 Hypertrophic cardiomyopathy in a cat. There is extreme hypertrophy of the myocardium, leading to near obliteration of each ventricular lumen and flattening of the interventricular septum.

hypertrophic cardiomyopathy may also be a sequel to hyper-thyroidism. Dietary taurine deficiency has also been implicated in the development of cardiomyopathy in cats.

Pericardial effusion

Pericardial effusion is not uncommon in the large and giant breeds of dog but is rare in cats. Ultrasound is the imaging modality of choice for the differentiation of pericardial effusion from cardiomegaly, and for investigating the cause of any pericardial effusion. Fluid is easily recognized as an echolucent band separating the epicardium and pericardium (Fig. 6.21). It has been shown experimentally in the dog that as little as 50 ml of saline in the pericardial sac can be detected ultra-sonographically. Any fluid will be distributed under the influence of gravity, so the position of the animal should be borne in mind when searching for fluid. Both epicardium and pericardium may appear thickened with echogenic tags and fronds in chronic cases. If a large amount of pericardial fluid is present, the heart often swings within it, giving rise to bizarre M mode traces.

When sufficient fluid is present to cause cardiac tamponnade, the effects on the right atrium and to a lesser extent the right ventricle may be noted. Both chambers may be compressed, but the right atrium may collapse completely during systole. If this is seen, it is an indication for immediate pericardial drainage.

Pericardial effusion in the dog may be idiopathic. A small pericardial effusion may be seen in association with congestive heart failure. However, pericardial effusion may also be associated with cardiac neoplasms, so a careful search should always be made for abnormal masses. The pericardial fluid surrounds and separates structures which facilitates identification of masses (Fig. 6.22). Neoplasms vary in size and shape, but are usually moderately echoic. Blood clots and thrombi within the right atrium and pericardial sac may mimic neoplasms. Ultrasound may help predict the surgical accessibility of any mass identified. Three main types of tumour are commonly associated with pericardial effusion:

1 Haemangiosarcoma. This usually arises from the right atrium so a meticulous search of the right atrial wall and lumen should be made.

2 Heart base tumour. These arise from the heart base in the region of the ascending aorta, but may extend in a number of

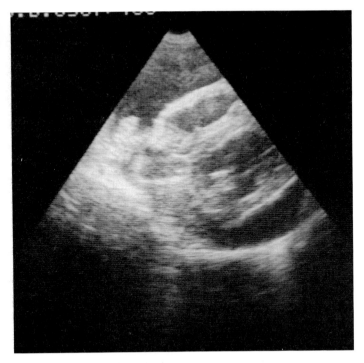

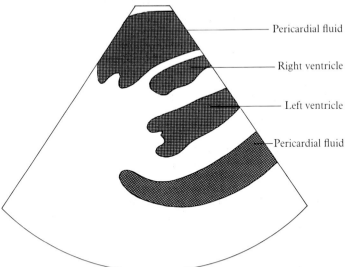

Pericardial fluid

Right ventricle

Left ventricle

Pericardial fluid

Fig. 6.21 Idiopathic pericardial effusion in an Old English Sheepdog. A large quantity of fluid surrounds the heart. No obvious mass could be seen in this or other views, and the effusion resolved after drainage.

directions and may invade the heart wall and chambers. Once again a careful examination of the heart from both sides of the thorax is necessary.

3 Mesothelioma. This is a diffuse tumour which may affect the epicardium, pericardium or pleura. Pleural and/or peri-

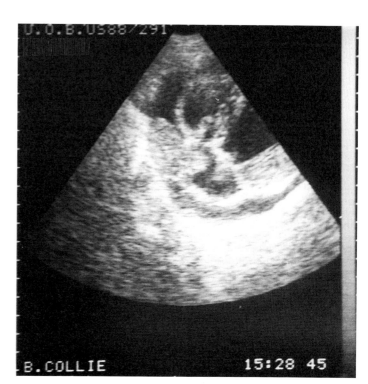

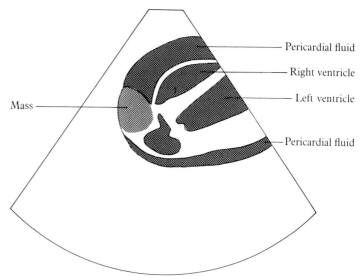

Pericardial fluid

Right ventricle

Left ventricle

Mass

Pericardial fluid

Fig. 6.22 Pericardial effusion in a Border Collie. In this case, a smooth, hypoechoic mass can be seen at the base of the heart, outlined by the pericardial fluid.

cardial fluid may result. Marked irregular thickening of the epicardium and/or pericardium should lead to consideration of this condition (Fig. 6.23), but chronic inflammatory change cannot be ruled out on the basis of ultrasound alone.

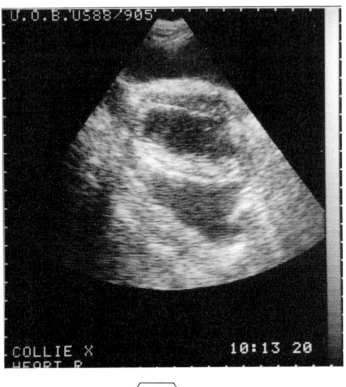

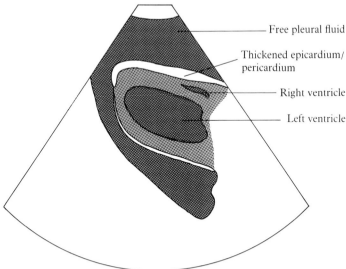

Free pleural fluid

Thickened epicardium/ pericardium

Right ventricle

Left ventricle

Fig. 6.23 Constrictive pericardial disease due to a mesothelioma in a cross-breed dog. A thick echogenic layer encases the heart and virtually obliterates the right ventricle. The free pleural fluid is due to right-sided heart failure.

Constrictive pericardial disease

This is a rare condition which can be difficult to diagnose. Ultrasonographically, a thickened, echogenic epicardium/

pericardium may be seen. Movement of the left ventricular free wall is restricted, leading to dampening of the M mode trace. Ventricular volumes may be normal or reduced. Paradoxical movement of the interventricular septum may be noted. Biatrial dilation can be seen.

Doppler techniques

Once again, it is beyond the scope of this book to consider Doppler techniques in any detail. However, Doppler ultrasound has much to offer in cardiac evaluation. The velocity of blood flow through the chambers of the heart and great vessels can be determined and thus, pressure gradients may be calculated. This is particularly useful in the diagnosis of ventricular outflow tract stenosis and allows an assessment of the functional severity of the lesion. Colour-flow techniques enable the direction and velocity of blood flow in the heart to be seen so that the competence of heart valves can be determined and the presence of abnormal shunting of blood shown.

Further reading

Bonagura, J.D. and Herring, D.S. (1985) Echocardiography: congenital heart disease. *Veterinary Clinics of North America: Small Animal Practice*, **15**, 1195–1208.

Bonagura, J.D. and Herring, D.S. (1985) Echocardiography: acquired heart disease. *Veterinary Clinics of North America: Small Animal Practice*, **15**, 1209–1224.

Bonagura, J.D. and Pipers, F.S. (1981) Echocardiographic features of pericardial effusion in dogs. *Journal of the American Veterinary Medical Association*, **179**, 49–56.

Bonagura, J.D. and Pipers, F.S. (1983) Diagnosis of cardiac lesions by contrast echocardiography. *Journal of the American Veterinary Medical Association*, **182**, 396–402.

Bonagura, J.D., O'Grady, M.R. and Herring, D.S. (1985) Echocardiography: principles of interpretation. *Veterinary Clinics of North America: Small Animal Practice*, **15**, 1177–1194.

Boon, J., Wingfield, W.E. and Miller, C.W. (1983) Echocardiographic indices in the normal dog. *Veterinary Radiology*, **24**, 214–221.

Lombard, C.W. (1984) Echocardiographic and clinical signs of canine dilated cardiomyopathy. *Journal of Small Animal Practice*, **25**, 59–70.

Lombard, C.W. and Buergelt, C.D. (1983) Vegetative bacterial endocarditis in dogs: echocardiographic diagnosis and clinical signs. *Journal of Small Animal Practice*, **24**, 325–339.

Soderberg, S.F., Boon, J.A., Wingfield, W.E. and Miller, C.W. (1983) M-mode echocardiography as a diagnostic aid for feline cardiomyopathy. *Veterinary Radiology*, **24**, 66–73.

Thomas, W.P. (1984) Two-dimensional real-time echocardiography in the dog: technique and anatomic validation. *Veterinary Radiology*, **25**, 50–64.

Thomas, W.P., Sisson, D., Bauer, T.G. and Reed, J.R. (1984) Detection of cardiac masses in dogs by 2-dimensional echocardiography. *Veterinary Radiology*, **25**, 65–72.

7/Imaging of the Thoracic Cavity

Imaging procedure

The structures within the thoracic cavity are not easy to image ultrasonographically since both the skeletal structures of the thoracic wall and air within the lungs prevent the passage of ultrasound. In order to avoid skeletal structures, the transducer may be placed between the ribs, behind the xiphisternum and angled cranially, or at the thoracic inlet and angled caudally. The precise transducer position selected will depend on the part of the thoracic cavity under examination. Once the acoustic window has been selected, hair should be clipped from the area and the skin prepared in a routine manner. Examination of the area of interest can then be carried out, using at least two different planes of section.

It is important to minimize the interference by air-filled lung by intelligent positioning of the animal. For example, it may be beneficial to place the animal in lateral recumbency with the affected side down, and to image from beneath. The position of the animal may also be varied according to the pathological changes expected. Free fluid, for example, will lie in the dependent parts of the thorax, while free air tends to rise to the uppermost parts. However, in cases of respiratory distress, the position of the animal may be limited to sternal recumbency, sitting or standing.

Normal appearance

The heart may be seen in the normal dog and cat when the transducer is placed in an intercostal position over the apex beat on the right or left thoracic wall. It can also sometimes be seen beyond the diaphragm from a xiphisternal approach. The diaphragm can be recognized as a thin echogenic line which moves with respiration. These structures act as useful landmarks within the thoracic cavity. However, in the normal dog and cat no other structures are usually identified. If the transducer is moved from the positions described above, only

150

interference from air-filled lung is seen. It may sometimes be possible to identify the great vessels of the cranial mediastinum when the transducer is placed at the thoracic inlet, but air within the trachea and occasionally within the oesophagus can interfere with image quality. Thus, ultrasonographic examination of the normal thorax is unrewarding, except for cardiac evaluation (see Chapter 6).

Abnormalities of the thorax

Free fluid within the thoracic cavity is readily identified ultrasonographically. Fluid tends to lie in the dependent portions of the thoracic cavity, so a meticulous search of these areas should be made if only a small amount of fluid is suspected. Larger quantities of fluid are usually easily seen, outlining and separating other thoracic structures (Fig. 7.1). It may on occasions be difficult to differentiate free thoracic and pericardial fluid. However, since pericardial fluid is contained, it should not move to the same extent as free thoracic fluid when the position of the animal is altered.

Free fluid is almost invariably anechoic irrespective of its nature (blood, chyle, transudate). The exception to this rule is purulent material, which may contain echoes depending on its consistency. If free fluid has been present in the pleural cavity for some time, thickening of the pleural and pericardial surfaces with echogenic tags and fronds may be seen. If there is sufficient reaction, loculated areas with trapped fluid may result.

Free air within the thoracic cavity is not easy to recognize ultrasonographically as it interferes with the image quality in just the same way as air-filled lung. Radiography is the imaging technique of choice for pneumothorax.

Masses within the pleural cavity may be identified ultrasonographically, depending on their size and position. Cranial mediastinal masses rarely cause clinical signs until they are quite large, and at this stage they are usually easy to image. When the transducer is moved cranial to the heart, the echopattern of solid tissue is seen rather than the normal lung interference pattern. There may be associated free fluid which further delineates the mass. Cranial mediastinal masses have a variable ultrasonographic appearance (Fig. 7.2). Thymic lymphosarcomata are often, but not invariably, homogeneous, hypoechoic and avascular. Masses of other histological types vary in echogenicity, architecture and vascularity. Irregular

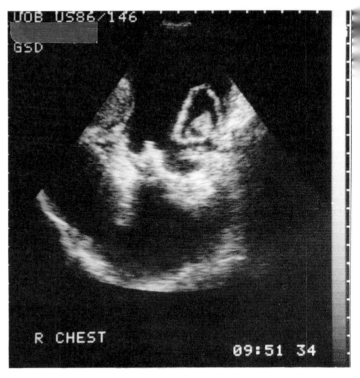

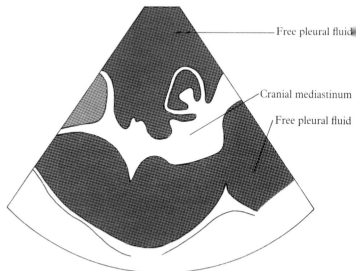

Free pleural fluid

Cranial mediastinum

Free pleural fluid

Fig. 7.1 Free thoracic fluid in a German Shepherd Dog. Membranes forming the cranial mediastinum are visible floating in the fluid.

anechoic patches represent areas of haemorrhage or necrosis, while bright echogenic areas represent fibrosis or calcification. A biopsy is usually required for a histological diagnosis.

Masses arising from or involving the thoracic wall can be

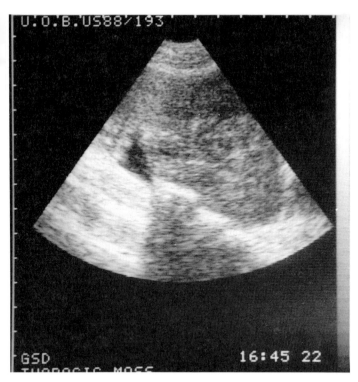

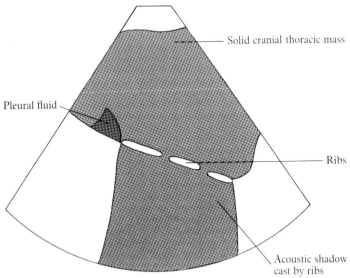

Solid cranial thoracic mass

Pleural fluid

Ribs

Acoustic shadow
cast by ribs

Fig. 7.2 Cranial mediastinal
mass in a German Shepherd
Dog. The mass is evenly
hypoechoic, which is typical of
lymphosarcoma. A small
amount of free fluid is visible.

examined ultrasonographically. Although swelling or deformity
is often detected on clinical examination, the full extent of the
mass may not be apparent until ultrasonography is performed.
The size of the intrathoracic portion of the mass and the

displacement or involvement of intrathoracic structures can be assessed, allowing a more informed prognosis to be given. However, the histological diagnosis cannot be ascertained from the ultrasonographic appearance alone.

Intrathoracic lymph nodes may enlarge due to lymphosarcoma or in association with other neoplastic or inflammatory disease. Enlargement of the retrosternal lymph node can be detected ultrasonographically as a mass in the cranioventral thorax above the first two or three sternebrae. The ultrasonographic appearance of the enlarged lymph node is non-specific — usually homogeneous and hypoechoic. Enlargement of the bronchial and mediastinal lymph nodes is not usually detected using conventional ultrasound as air-filled lung lies on either side. Endoscopic ultrasound may allow evaluation of these lymph nodes, but this technique is not yet widely available.

Pulmonary changes cannot be evaluated accurately using ultrasound. Because of the image interference caused by air, subtle changes in the pulmonary vasculature, bronchial tree, alveoli and interstitium are not seen. Radiography is consequently the imaging technique of choice. However, large areas of pulmonary consolidation located peripherally may be appreciated ultrasonographically as irregular masses of mild–moderate echogenicity (Fig. 7.3). If the bronchi are fluid-filled, then anechoic channels may be seen within these masses. More often there is still air within the bronchi or in small clusters of alveoli, leading to echogenic spots with acoustic shadowing. Intrapulmonary masses may also be imaged if they are peripherally located (Fig. 7.4). This may on occasions be useful as it is possible to determine whether a mass is solid (e.g. neoplasm, granuloma), irregularly cavitating (e.g. necrotic neoplasm, abscess) or smooth and fluid-filled (e.g. haematocyst). Ultrasound may be used to guide a needle into a mass for aspiration or biopsy.

Thoracic ultrasonography may be particularly useful in cases of rupture of the diaphragm. When the tear is left-sided, the stomach and/or small intestine commonly move into the thoracic cavity. Ultrasonography may demonstrate displacement of the heart away from the left thoracic wall by tissue of heterogeneous echogenicity. Such cases are, however, more easily recognized radiographically. When the tear is right-sided, part of the liver may pass into the thoracic cavity. These cases are difficult to diagnose radiographically, particularly if hepatic incarceration leads to thoracic effusion. Using

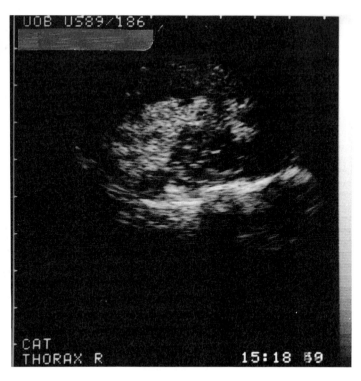

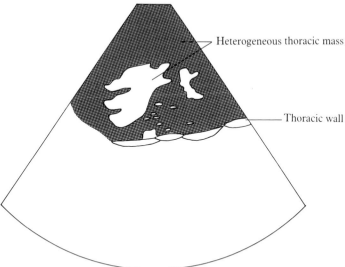

Heterogeneous thoracic mass

Thoracic wall

Fig. 7.3 Inflammatory pulmonary consolidation in a cat. A heterogeneous solid mass is seen instead of the normal acoustic shadows of air-filled lung.

ultrasound, the intrathoracic portion of the liver is easily recognized adjacent to, and sometimes displacing, the heart (Fig. 7.5). The presence of fluid highlights the entrapped viscus. It is important to remember that if the transducer is

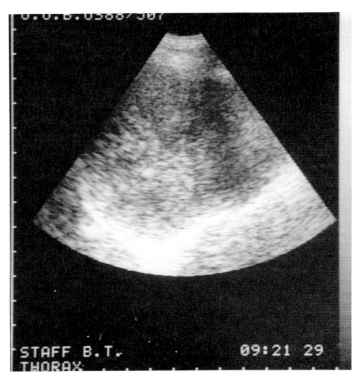

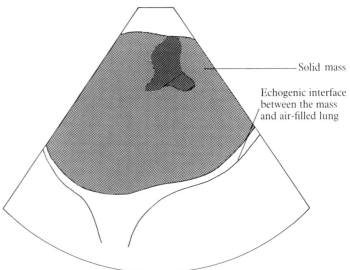

Solid mass

Echogenic interface
between the mass
and air-filled lung

Fig. 7.4 Pulmonary neoplasm
in a Staffordshire Bull Terrier.
A solid, slightly heterogeneous
mass abuts the thoracic wall.

placed behind the xiphisternum and angled cranially, mirror
image artefacts frequently give rise to the illusion of liver
beyond the diaphragm in normal dogs and cats. To be confi-
dent that part of the liver is intrathoracic, this must be

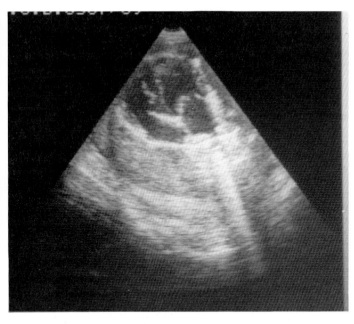

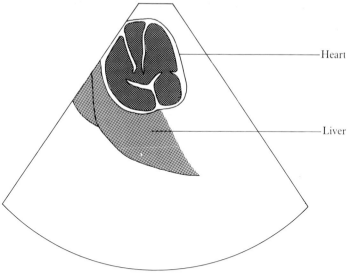

Heart

Liver

Fig. 7.5 Rupture of the diaphragm in a Border Collie. The transducer has been placed on the left thoracic wall, showing a four chamber view of the heart and a parenchymatous organ (liver) between the heart and the right thoracic wall.

confirmed with the transducer placed in an intercostal position.

Peritoneo-pericardial hernia is a congenital anomaly which results in abdominal viscera passing into the pericardial sac. Ultrasonographically, abdominal organs are easily recognized in the thoracic cavity, but it may be difficult to be sure they are in the pericardial sac rather than free in the thoracic cavity. Thus, it can be difficult to differentiate a congenital peritoneo-pericardial hernia and a traumatic diaphragmatic rupture ultrasonographically, although the history may help clarify the situation.

In summary, ultrasonographic evaluation of the thorax is often useful in the presence of fluid and/or intrathoracic masses. It must, however, always be used in conjunction with radiography as pulmonary disease and abnormalities of mediastinal structures are rarely detected ultrasonographically.

8/Imaging of the Eye

Imaging procedure

A high-frequency transducer (7.5−10 MHz) is essential to produce diagnostic images of the eye and retrobulbar tissues. The sound beam is required to penetrate only a few centimetres of tissue, but image detail is of paramount importance.

It may be useful to sedate the animal prior to ultrasonographic examination of the eye, depending on its temperament. However, it is a procedure that is surprisingly well-tolerated by most dogs and cats. If the eye is very painful, topical local anaesthesia may make the examination more comfortable. Alternatively, light general anaesthesia may be combined with topical local anaesthesia.

The examination may be carried out with the patient in a sitting or standing position, but the animal should be restrained from backing away. The head should be held firmly but gently and the eyelids held apart. In the cat, the third eyelid often moves to cover the eye as the transducer approaches. In such instances the transducer may be positioned on the third eyelid. This does not usually occur in the dog, so the transducer is placed directly on the cornea (Fig. 8.1). Gentle pressure may be applied to maintain good contact between the transducer and the cornea, but care should be taken not to lacerate or abrade the corneal surface. Most commercial gels are water soluble and non-irritant and may be used safely in the eye. Depending on the focal zone of the transducer used, it may be necessary to use a stand-off between the transducer and cornea. This is particularly helpful for critical evaluation of the anterior chamber and lens.

It is possible to examine the eye through the closed eyelids although image quality is not as good. The lids are hairy in the dog and cat, but it is generally impractical to clip this area. It is therefore important to use liberal quantities of acoustic gel.

The eye should be examined first in horizontal section with the plane of the sound beam running from medial to lateral

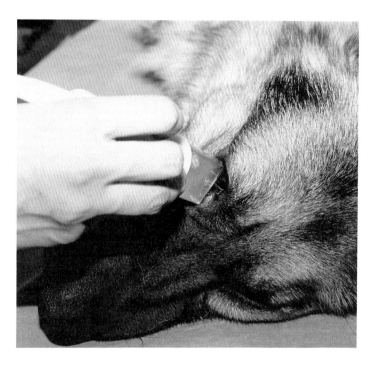

Fig. 8.1 Imaging the eye.

canthus. Sweeps of the beam should be made dorsally and ventrally to ensure that the globe and retrobulbar tissues are thoroughly examined. The head of the transducer should then be rotated through 90° to image a vertical section of the eye. Sweeps of the beam should be made medially and laterally.

It is useful to examine both eyes even if only one is abnormal. The unaffected eye may be used as a reference for normal size, shape and anatomy in that individual.

When the ultrasound examination has been completed, excess acoustic gel should be carefully wiped from the eyes.

Normal appearance

The normal eye is a smooth, well-circumscribed, rounded structure with anechoic contents (Fig. 8.2). Both the aqueous and the vitreous humour should be completely anechoic although reverberation artefacts may sometimes give rise to spurious echoes. Artefactual echoes should disappear when the plane of section is changed while true echoes arising from pathological changes in the eye should remain consistent.

The cornea is not clearly demarcated unless a stand-off is used. It is a smooth echogenic layer. The lens has curved

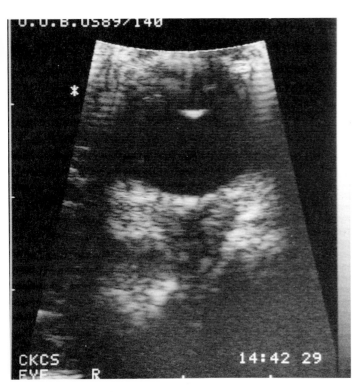

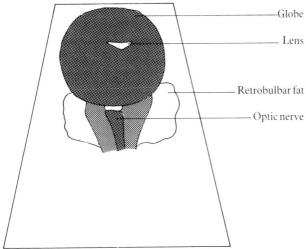

Fig. 8.2   Normal eye in a
Cavalier King Charles Spaniel.

anterior and posterior surfaces which produce scattered reflections, so it is usual to see echoes from the central part of the
lens only, where the incident sound beam is perpendicular to
the reflecting surface. The ciliary body may be seen as small,
moderately echoic masses on each side of the lens. The separate

layers comprising the back of the globe (the retina, choroid and sclera) are not usually seen as individual entities but as a single echogenic curved line. The slightly recessed area of the head of the optic nerve may be identified.

The retrobulbar tissues are of moderate echogenicity because of the presence of large amounts of fat. They normally form an orderly cone behind the eye. The optic nerve may be recognized as a hypoechoic channel coursing ventromedially towards the back of the orbit. It may also sometimes be possible to define individual extraocular muscles, which are also hypoechoic, within the retrobulbar tissues.

Abnormalities of the third eyelid and periocular tissues

Abnormalities of the third eyelid and periocular tissues are generally detected on clinical examination. If a mass is present which prevents examination of the eye, ultrasound may be used to assess the presence or absence of ocular involvement (Fig. 8.3). This facilitates an informed decision regarding treatment and prognosis.

Abnormalities of the eye

Many abnormalities of the eye can be diagnosed by means of clinical and ophthalmoscopic examinations. However, in situations where visual examination of the eye is impossible, ultrasonography may provide valuable information. Thus ultrasonograhic examination of the eye may be useful in animals with masses of the third eyelid or periocular tissues, corneal or lenticular opacity, or hyphaema.

An alteration in the size of the globe may be noted in certain conditions, e.g. hydrophthalmos, microphthalmos, phthisis bulbi. Although such changes are generally apparent on clinical examination, ultrasound allows accurate measurement of the size of the eye and quantitative evaluation of change over a period of time. The normal ultrasonographic dimensions of the eye in a group of mixed breed dogs of similar body weight have been reported. The breed standards however, determine the size of the eye which is considered normal in pure-bred dogs, and this may vary considerably between breeds. In unilateral conditions, therefore, it is more useful to use the normal eye as a standard for that individual.

The lens normally produces only scattered echoes from its anterior and posterior surfaces. A cataractous lens has in-

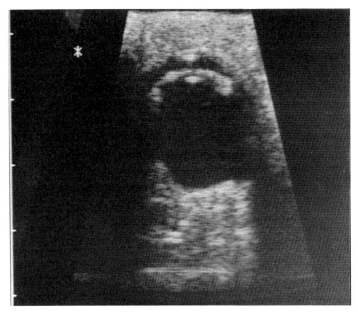

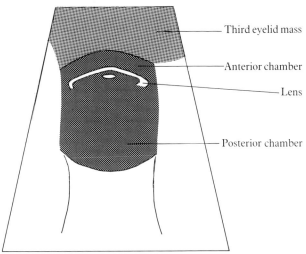

Third eyelid mass

Anterior chamber

Lens

Posterior chamber

Fig. 8.3 Third eyelid mass in a Welsh Springer Spaniel. The anterior chamber of the eye and the lens are more clearly seen than usual, beyond the third eyelid mass. The globe is ultrasonographically normal.

creased echogenicity, and it is usual to see the entire outline of the lens (Fig. 8.4). Luxation of the lens into the anterior or posterior chambers or displacement of the lens by an intraocular mass may be readily identified (Fig. 8.4).

Intraocular masses are of variable ultrasonographic appearance but are usually of mild–moderate echogenicity. The extent of the mass within the globe and the involvement of periocular tissues may be evaluated, allowing a rational treat-

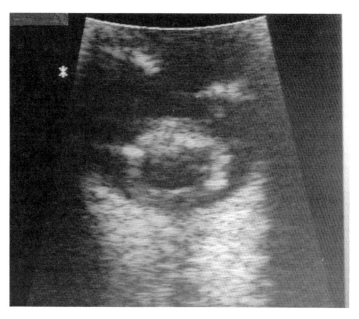

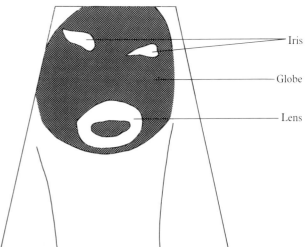

Iris

Globe

Lens

Fig. 8.4 Posterior dislocation
of the lens in a Weimaraner.
The lens is lying in an
abnormal position in the
posterior chamber. In this case,
the lens is also cataractous, and
so has a particularly echogenic
outline.

ment to be instituted. However, the histological nature of
such masses cannot be determined using ultrasonographic
criteria alone.

Haemorrhage within the eye gives rise to echoes in the
appropriate chamber. Once clotting has occurred, irregular
hypoechoic masses may be seen which are indistinguishable
from other soft tissue masses (Fig. 8.5). The gradual resolution
of changes supports a diagnosis of intraocular haemorrhage,
but in cases where haemorrhage is recurrent it may be im-

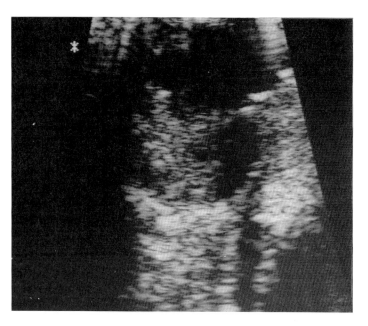

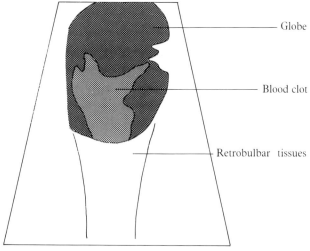

— Globe

— Blood clot

— Retrobulbar tissues

Fig. 8.5 Intraocular
haemorrhage in a Corgi. An
irregular mass of moderate
echogenicity in the posterior
chamber represents a blood
clot.

possible to differentiate blood clots and neoplasms. Endo-
phthalmitis may also give rise to echoes within the anterior
and/or posterior chambers of the eye, because of pus formation.

Intraocular foreign bodies may be detected if they are large
enough but a meticulous examination of the whole globe is
essential. Most foreign materials are echogenic and cast a
clear acoustic shadow. Metallic foreign bodies are also echogenic but may cast a stream of reverberations rather than a
shadow. Small foreign bodies, such as thorns, are easily missed.

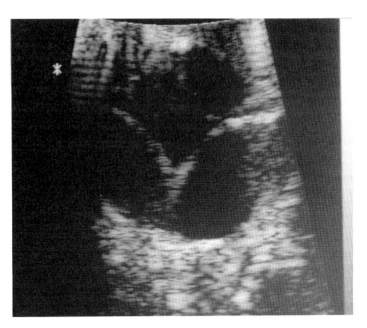

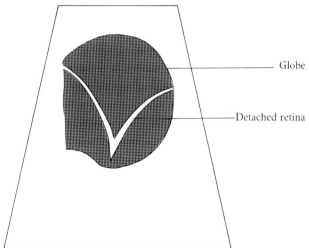

Globe

Detached retina

Fig. 8.6 Retinal detachment in a Corgi. The retina is completely detached, held only at the optic disc and the ciliary body.

Retinal detachment may be diagnosed ultrasonographically. The detached portion of retina is seen as a linear echogenicity raised from the wall of the globe and separated from it by fluid. In cases of complete retinal detachment, a characteristic echogenic 'V' is seen in the posterior chamber, representing the retina attached only at the optic disc and the ciliary body (Fig. 8.6). Small focal areas of retinal detachment may be overlooked.

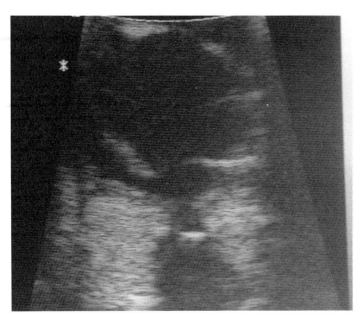

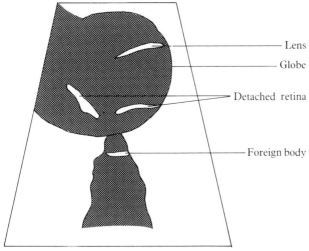

Lens

Globe

Detached retina

Foreign body

Fig. 8.7 Retrobulbar foreign body in a cat. The echogenic foreign body in the retrobulbar tissues casts an acoustic shadow. Note also the retinal detachment, which is due to passage of the foreign body through the globe.

Abnormalities of the retrobulbar tissues

Ultrasound is the imaging technique of choice for the retro-bulbar area. Foreign bodies, whether radiolucent or radiodense, may be detected and accurately localized using ultrasound. As previously mentioned, most foreign bodies appear echogenic, casting an acoustic shadow or a stream of reverberations (Fig. 8.7).

Retrobulbar masses may be identified ultrasonographically. In small animals, such masses are usually either neoplasms or abscesses. Abscesses are often rather poorly defined and of mixed echogenicity, although the ultrasonographic appearance may be variable. Neoplasms may also vary greatly in echogenicity and homogeneity. It may therefore not be possible to differentiate an abscess and a neoplasm on ultrasonographic criteria alone, although the history and clinical examination may be helpful. In cases of uncertainty, ultrasound may be used to localize the mass accurately and to guide a needle into the area for aspiration or biopsy.

Safety of ophthalmic ultrasound

There have been published reports of ocular damage in rabbits exposed to high intensity or long duration ultrasound. The effects noted include corneal opacification, cataract formation, vitreal liquefaction, and choroid oedema and necrosis. However, the levels of ultrasound used for diagnostic purposes have no known adverse effects in man or animals. Although care must be taken when the transducer is placed on the surface of the cornea, ophthalmic ultrasound may be used as a safe and painless diagnostic technique.

Further reading

Dziezyc, J. and Hager, D.A. (1988) Ocular ultrasonography in veterinary medicine. *Seminars in Veterinary Medicine and Surgery (Small Animal)*, 3, 1–9.
Dziezyc, J., Hager, D.A. and Millichamp, N.J. (1987) Two-dimensional real-time ocular ultrasonography in the diagnosis of ocular lesions in dogs. *Journal of the American Animal Hospitals Association*, 23, 501–508.
Eisenberg, H.M. (1985) Ultrasonography of the eye and orbit. *Veterinary Clinics of North America: Small Animal Practice*, 15, 1263–1274.
Hager, D.A., Dziezyc, J. and Millichamp, N.J. (1987) Two-dimensional real-time ocular ultrasonography in the dog: technique and normal anatomy. *Veterinary Radiology*, 28, 60–65.
Miller, W.W. and Carter, R.E. (1985) B-scan ultrasonography for the detection of space-occupying ocular masses. *Journal of the American Veterinary Medical Association*, 187, 66–68.
Schiffer, S.P., Rantanen, N.W., Leary, G.A. and Bryan, G.M. (1982) Biometric study of the eye using A-mode ultrasonography. *American Journal of Veterinary Research*, 43, 826–830.

9/Imaging of other Superficial Soft Tissues

Imaging procedure

Any of the superficial soft tissues of small animals may be imaged ultrasonographically. The hair over the area should be clipped and the skin prepared routinely. In most instances a high-frequency transducer (7.5–10 MHz) should be selected as the tissue penetration required is minimal. A stand-off may be necessary to allow examination of very superficial structures. Occasionally, the thickness of soft tissues under examination is such that a medium frequency transducer (3.5–5 MHz) must be used to give adequate tissue penetration.

The area of interest should then be imaged in at least two planes of section, taking care to sweep through the whole region. When the superficial soft tissues of the limbs are under examination, it is always useful to image the normal contralateral limb. This allows a reference of the normal ultrasonographic anatomy of the area to be obtained. The same principle applies when examining regions of the head, neck or trunk away from the midline.

Superficial masses

Ultrasound may be used to characterize the nature of superficial masses. Clearly, the history and clinical examination are invaluable, and frequently ultrasound will add no extra information. In some cases however, ultrasound may be useful in determining whether a mass is homogeneous or heterogeneous in architecture, whether it is predominantly solid or fluid-filled, and whether it is encapsulated or locally infiltrative. It may also be important to discover prior to surgery whether a mass surrounds or invades major blood vessels in the region, and whether the mass itself contains obvious large blood vessels.

Benign superficial neoplasms are usually clearly circumscribed with no invasion of surrounding tissues. Superficial lipomata often have a characteristic texture on palpation, but this is by no means always the case. Lipomata located more deeply between or beneath muscle layers may be particularly difficult to characterize on palpation. However, lipomata have a typical ultrasonographic appearance of a well-circumscribed, homogeneous, moderately echoic mass with echogenic spots scattered throughout (Fig. 9.1). Other benign neoplasms vary in their ultrasonographic appearance.

Malignant superficial neoplasms also have a very variable ultrasonographic architecture. Large masses in particular are often heterogeneous, with anechoic areas of necrosis and haemorrhage, and echogenic patches representing fibrosis and calcification. Most malignant neoplasms are poorly circumscribed, with no clear boundaries between normal and abnormal tissue (Fig. 9.2). It is not possible, however, to determine the histological type of most neoplasms by the ultrasonographic appearance alone.

Potentially, ultrasound may be used for the detection of small impalpable masses. For example, the area of the thyroid may be searched ultrasonographically in cats or dogs showing clinical and biochemical evidence of hyperthyroidism or, more rarely, primary hyperparathyroidism. However, the sensitivity and specificity of ultrasound used in this way remains to be evaluated.

Not all superficial masses in small animals are neoplastic — haematomata and abscesses also commonly occur. Haematomata may show a variable ultrasonographic pattern depending on the age of the lesion and the stages of clotting and organization present. Such masses should, however, slowly resolve with time. Superficial abscesses which are filled with pus are usually obvious clinically. Deeper abscesses with ramifying tracts, pockets of pus and granulation tissue may be less obvious. Ultrasonographically, these abscesses appear poorly circumscribed and heterogeneous with multiple hypo/anechoic pockets (Fig. 9.3). This appearance is non-specific and can be seen also in necrotic tumours and haematomata.

The major potential benefit of ultrasonographic examination of persistent abscesses is that foreign bodies may be detected and accurately localized prior to surgical exploration. Most foreign bodies (sticks and splinters, glass, tooth, bone) should cast clear acoustic shadows (Fig. 9.4). Metallic foreign bodies are usually intensely echogenic and may cast a stream of reverberations rather than an acoustic shadow. However, present experience indicates that the ubiquitous grass seed remains

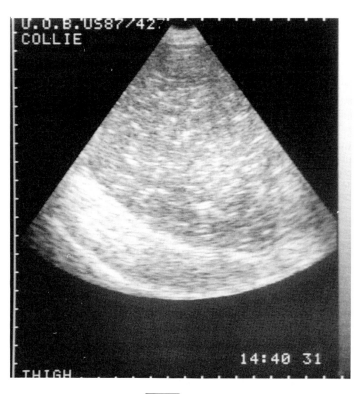

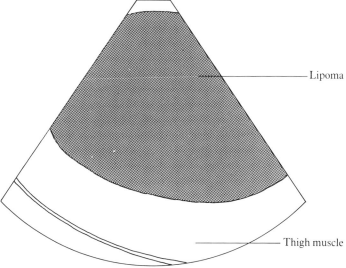

— Lipoma

— Thigh muscle

Fig. 9.1 Lipoma in a Border Collie. The mass is well-circumscribed with a speckled texture.

difficult, if not impossible, to detect. When searching for foreign bodies within an abscess it is important to identify normal anatomical structures which may cast shadows. In the neck, for example, the bodies and transverse processes of the

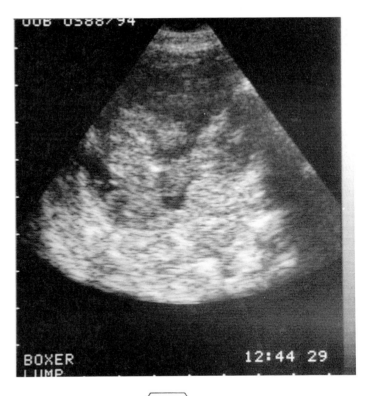

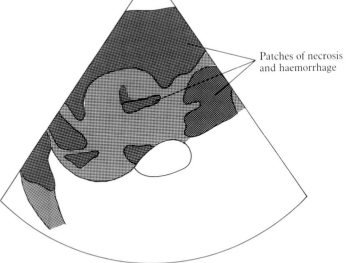

Patches of necrosis
and haemorrhage

Fig. 9.2 Thyroid carcinoma
in a Boxer. The mass is very
poorly defined with no clear
boundaries. Irregular anechoic
and hypoechoic areas probably
represent patches of necrosis or
haemorrhage.

cervical vertebrae, the hyoid apparatus and the trachea may
all cast acoustic shadows. In addition, tracts discharging to
the surface may contain air which gives rise to shadowing.

Sialocoeles are readily identifiable ultrasonographically.

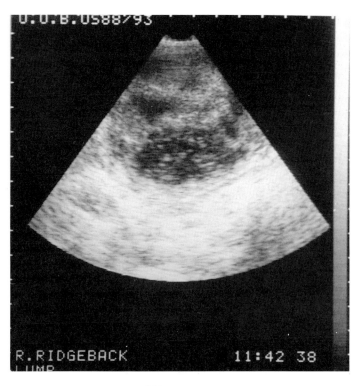

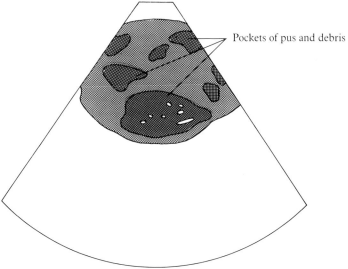

Pockets of pus and debris

Fig. 9.3 Abscess in a Rhodesian Ridgeback. The mass is poorly defined, and contains multiple, irregular, anechoic patches representing fluid and necrotic tissue.

They are well-circumscribed structures filled with fluid which usually contains some echoes (Fig. 9.5). They can be differentiated from homogeneous solid masses such as enlarged lymph nodes since the echoes swirl about when the mass is

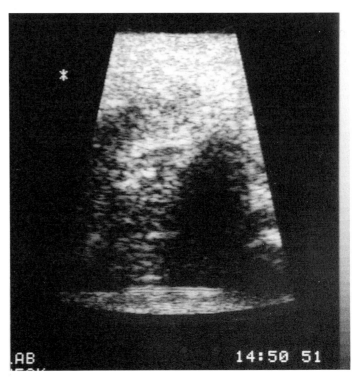

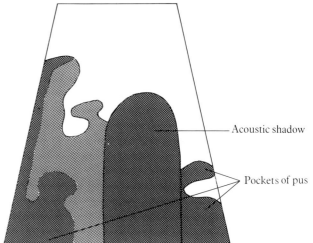

Fig. 9.4 Foreign body abscess in a Labrador. The abscess is seen as an area of heterogeneous echogenicity with no clear boundaries. There is an area within this of strong acoustic shadowing, which is due to a stick foreign body.

ballotted. Occasionally, the salivary gland may be seen adjacent to the fluid collection. However, sialocoeles are not usually difficult to diagnose clinically, and since ultrasound can rarely identify the particular gland involved, it adds little useful information.

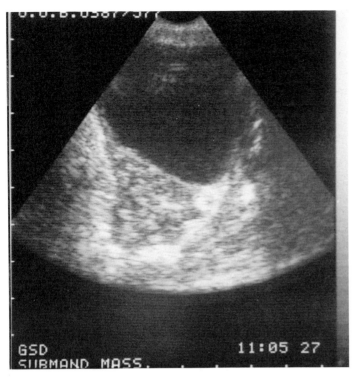

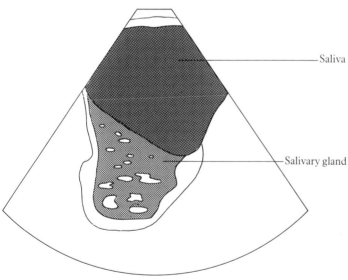

Saliva

Salivary gland

Fig. 9.5 Sialocoele in a German Shepherd Dog. The fluid collection is well-circumscribed. The irregular mass of heterogeneous echogenicity adjacent to the fluid is probably salivary gland.

Tendons

Ultrasound may be used to evaluate the tendons of the distal limbs in order to assess injury and to monitor subsequent

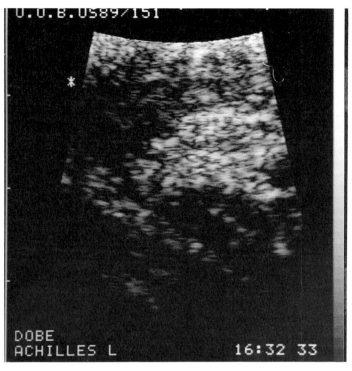

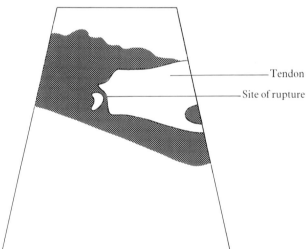

Tendon
Site of rupture

Fig. 9.6 Rupture of the Achilles tendon in a Doberman. The site of rupture, close to the musculotendinous junction, can be clearly seen.

healing. A high-resolution transducer (10 MHz) is essential if adequate detail is to be seen. Even so, the small branches of the flexor and extensor tendons distal to the carpus and hock are difficult to examine. The larger tendons, such as the achilles tendon, can be more accurately assessed.

It may be possible to detect total or partial rupture of a tendon (Fig. 9.6). Less severe injuries to the tendons may theoretically be identified by disruption of normal fibre alignment and/or thickening of the tendon, but the sensitivity of ultrasound in the detection of tendon injuries in small animals has yet to be evaluated. Ultrasound may also be useful in demonstrating fluid within the tendon sheath in cases of septic or sterile tenosynovitis. A distinct anechoic band is seen surrounding and separating tendinous structures.

10/Ultrasound-guided Biopsy Techniques

Throughout the preceding chapters, the ultrasonographic changes which may be seen associated with lesions of the soft tissues of the body have been described. It has been emphasized that the changes seen are often non-specific. In addition, diffuse inflammatory or infiltrative diseases of the parenchymal organs may not result in any ultrasonographic abnormality. Cytological or histological examination is therefore frequently indicated if a definitive diagnosis is required. Samples of fluid or soft tissues may be collected during exploratory surgery of the thoracic or abdominal cavities. In many instances, however, percutaneous sampling techniques may be preferred as these are less traumatic and can often be performed under sedation and local anaesthesia.

Ultrasound can be used to watch the needle as it is introduced percutaneously into the thoracic or abdominal cavities. The needle may then be directed precisely into the organ of interest. Continuous real-time ultrasonographic monitoring of the position of the needle minimizes the risks associated with percutaneous sampling techniques, such as inadvertent puncture of major blood vessels or adjacent organs. In addition, the diagnostic yield is maximized as the needle can be placed accurately in the organ of interest, and even in small focal lesions within an organ.

Aspiration or core biopsy?

Free fluid within a body cavity or fluid contained within a viscus may be aspirated using a syringe and fine gauge needle. Cytological, biochemical and bacteriological examination of the fluid may then be undertaken. Fine needle aspirates of soft tissues may be obtained in a similar way and the resulting sample examined cytologically. Cytology is a sensitive method of detecting malignancy but tissue architecture cannot be evaluated. This limits its application in the characterization of benign and certain well-differentiated malignant lesions.

More commonly, a core biopsy of soft tissues is collected,

allowing histological examination of the sample. Conventionally, core biopsies have been obtained using large gauge (20 G or larger) needles specifically designed for the purpose. More recently, fine needle biopsies using needles with an outer diameter of less than 1 mm (smaller than 20 G) have proved to be useful. Whichever technique is selected, it should be appreciated that the larger the sample collected, the more likely it is that a firm diagnosis will be possible. In addition, a fine needle is inevitably more flexible than a needle of larger calibre and so may be more readily deflected within the body. However, the risks associated with percutaneous biopsy are likely to increase with large calibre needles. The author has most commonly used 18 G needles for ultrasound guided percutaneous biopsy of parenchymal organs and solid masses. To date the diagnostic quality of the samples has been good and there have been no major complications.

Biopsy needles

A large variety of types of biopsy needle are available, and the advantages and disadvantages of each design have been well-documented. They fall into two main categories: the cutting type (e.g. Tru-Cut, Vim-Silverman); and the aspiration type (e.g. Menghini, Chiba). The needle selected will depend largely on availability and personal preference, but it is worth considering whether one or two hands are required to collect the sample. If the needle can be operated with one hand, a single person can manipulate the transducer and the biopsy needle. It is important that the operator becomes thoroughly familiar with the mechanism of action of the biopsy needle selected before attempting a percutaneous biopsy in a living animal.

An automatic spring-loaded biopsy device is also available ('Biopty TM', Radiplast). This uses a Tru-Cut type needle but can be operated with one hand. The biopsy action is very quick and precise so that the sample obtained is usually of good quality and the procedure is relatively painless. The needles are available in two sizes only (18 G and 14 G).

Whichever type of biopsy needle is chosen, it can usually be identified ultrasonographically as long as it remains in the plane of the sound beam. The needle is echogenic, but it is often easier to detect the movement of tissues as the needle passes through them than the needle itself. Various modifications in needle design have been suggested to increase the echogenicity and thus the visibility of the needle. These involve roughening or scoring part of the outer surface of the needle or inserting a scored stylet inside the needle to increase sound reflection. A simpler technique of enhancing visualization of the tip of the needle involves injection of a small amount of air (0.3−0.5 ml) via the biopsy needle. The air will emerge at the tip of the needle and will be intensely echogenic. Such manipulations are, however, rarely required.

Introduction of the biopsy needle

It is possible to introduce the biopsy needle freehand adjacent to the transducer (Fig. 10.1). It is important to ensure that the needle remains in the plane of the sound beam because otherwise it will not be seen on the display screen. The major advantage of the freehand technique is that no specialized equipment is required. There is also flexibility in the positioning and direction of the needle. However, it may be difficult to see the needle.

Alternatively, the biopsy needle may be introduced via a guide hole. There are special biopsy transducers available which incorporate a central canal or slot for introduction of the needle. More commonly, a clip-on needle guide can be attached to the transducer, allowing the needle to be introduced adjacent to the transducer (Fig. 10.2). The main advantage of such guides is that they ensure that the needle remains in the plane of the beam, so that seeing the needle on the screen is rarely a problem. The disadvantages are that the guides may be too bulky for use in small dogs and cats, and there are limitations in both the gauge of needle which can be used and the angle of introduction of the needle. It is probably easier to use a guide while learning ultrasound guided biopsy techniques, but with experience a freehand technique may be preferred.

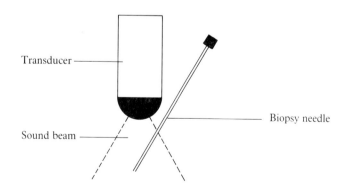

Fig. 10.1 'Freehand' biopsy technique. The needle is introduced adjacent to the transducer, in the same plane as the sound beam.

Transducer

Sound beam

Biopsy needle

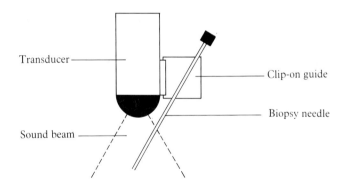

Transducer

Clip-on guide

Biopsy needle

Sound beam

Fig. 10.2 Biopsy technique using a clip-on guide. The needle is introduced through the channel in the guide.

Many ultrasound machines now have software which allows display of the projected needle path on the screen. The projected path clearly only applies if the appropriate needle guide is used, but may be useful in positioning and detecting the needle when the technique is being learnt.

The procedure for ultrasound-guided biopsy

A thorough clinical examination and diagnostic evaluation of the animal should be completed before a percutaneous biopsy is undertaken. The animal must also be assessed for any abnormalities in haemostasis by checking whole blood clotting time, prothrombin time, partial thromboplastin time and platelet numbers. Abnormalities in blood clotting do not necessarily constitute an absolute contraindication to percutaneous biopsy of internal organs, but the increased risks of significant haemorrhage should be considered.

It is vital that the animal remains reasonably still during the biopsy procedure as sudden movements can lead to laceration of blood vessels and organs. Therefore, it is usually wise to sedate the animal. The incorporation of an analgesic in the sedation protocol is useful as this will alleviate any discomfort during and after the biopsy procedure. If the animal is particularly uncooperative or the biopsy site is unusually painful, general anaesthesia may be indicated.

After sedation or induction of general anaesthesia, the animal is positioned for ultrasonographic examination of the appropriate organ. If the animal is conscious, particular care should be taken to ensure that it is comfortable, in order to minimize voluntary movements. The organ which is to be biopsied should be examined ultrasonographically to ensure that any lesions are still clearly visible and to allow estimation of the point of entry of the biopsy needle.

The clipped area of skin should then be cleaned thoroughly and prepared aseptically. If the animal is conscious, local anaesthetic should be infiltrated into the skin, subcutaneous tissues and thoracic or abdominal wall at the site of needle puncture. A small nick in the skin made with a scalpel blade at this site facilitates passage of the needle. In general it is preferable to cover the transducer with a sterile sleeve and to use sterile gel on the skin surface to achieve good transducer contact. Sterile sleeves and gel are commercially available — alternatively small packs of standard ultrasound gel can be sterilized as required in an autoclave and the transducer covered with a sterile surgical glove. If a clip-on needle guide is used, this should be attached to the covered transducer and should clearly also be sterile. Maintenance of sterility of the skin surface, transducer, needle guide and needle minimizes the risk of introducing infection into the body cavities. It has been reported however that thorough cleaning of the transducer is quite adequate without the addition of a sterile transducer cover.

Once the site and equipment have been prepared, the organ of interest is imaged in the optimal plane for the proposed biopsy. The biopsy needle may then be introduced, either freehand or through a needle guide, through the nick in the skin and into the appropriate body cavity. The needle tip can be watched on the screen and directed towards the site of interest. When the needle tip is in the correct position, the biopsy or aspirate may be taken and the needle withdrawn.

The number of biopsy attempts in each patient will vary according to the size of samples obtained and the cooperation of the dog or cat. In the Langford House clinic, the number of biopsies per organ on a single occasion is usually restricted to two, although on rare occasions a third attempt will be made if the first two attempts have proved unsatisfactory.

A careful ultrasonographic examination of the organ should be made after the biopsy procedure to check for significant haemorrhage. The needle tract often remains visible for some time after withdrawal of the needle from parenchymatous organs, due to minor intraparenchymal haemorrhage.

After completion of the biopsy, the animal should be allowed to recover quietly for 24—48 h. A close watch should be kept for evidence of significant intracavitary haemorrhage for the first 4—6 h. Abdominal palpation should be avoided where possible during the recovery period as this may precipitate or prolong haemorrhage from the biopsy site.

Complications of percutaneous biopsy

The general complications of percutaneous needle biopsy include haemorrhage, damage to adjacent tissues, and seeding of tumour cells along the biopsy tract. Mild transient discomfort is experienced by most human patients, with pain persisting for some hours in a few individuals. In addition, complications specific to the biopsy of certain organs have been described and are noted below.

In a large series of fine needle abdominal biopsies in man, the incidence of mortality was 0.008%. Major complications (biliary peritonitis, tumour seeding, intrahepatic haematoma and peritonitis) developed in 0.05% of patients and minor complications in 0.49%. Although a larger needle theoretically increases the risk of complications, these risks are minimized under the controlled conditions of ultrasound guidance.

Using the general principles of ultrasound guidance outlined above, it is theoretically possible to collect fluid or tissue samples from any thoracic or abdominal structure which can be clearly imaged. The risks of the procedure in each case should be weighed against the potential clinical benefit. The indications for percutaneous biopsy of the liver, kidney and prostate in small animals are relatively common. Points pertinent to the biopsy of these specific organs are outlined below.

Liver biopsy

Percutaneous biopsy of the liver is a reasonably straightforward procedure when performed under ultrasound guidance. The dog or cat is usually placed in dorsal recumbency and the liver imaged with the transducer placed behind the xiphisternum. The needle may then be introduced adjacent to the transducer and directed into the appropriate part of the liver. Occasionally the liver is so small that it can only be imaged with the animal lying in left lateral recumbency and the transducer placed between the ribs. The needle can then be introduced intercostally.

It is important that the animal is starved for 8–12 h prior to biopsy of the liver. This ensures an empty stomach, which maximizes the visibility of the liver and minimizes the chances of puncturing the stomach with the needle. However, starvation usually also results in a full gall bladder. It is vital to avoid puncturing the gall bladder as this may lead to bile peritonitis — a serious complication which may prove fatal. A small quantity of fat given orally 30–60 min before the biopsy procedure may stimulate gall bladder contraction and emptying, but often seems to have little effect. However, if care is taken to identify the gall bladder on the preliminary scan, it should not be difficult to avoid it when introducing the biopsy needle. To minimize the risk of post biopsy haemorrhage, the biopsy site should ideally be deep within the liver parenchyma (Fig. 10.3).

Contraindications for biopsy of the liver include abnormalities of blood clotting, severe hepatic venous congestion and extrahepatic biliary obstruction (bile subjected to abnormally high intraductal pressure can escape along the biopsy tract into the peritoneal cavity resulting in bile peritonitis). The presence of ascites has been considered a contraindication to percutaneous biopsy of the liver in the past because of the risks of uncontrolled haemorrhage or leakage of ascitic fluid from the abdominal cavity. However, a study in man showed no significant difference in the complication rate in patients with and without ascites. Ascites should not, therefore, be considered a contraindication to liver biopsy, but may make the biopsy procedure technically more difficult. The liver lobes tend to float away from the needle tip and the distance the needle must be introduced is increased. However, the visibility of the needle is enhanced by the fluid.

Kidney biopsy

Percutaneous renal biopsies are usually performed under general anaesthesia rather than sedation and local anaesthesia. The reason for this is that the kidney is a highly vascular organ and uncontrolled movements of the animal can lead to renal laceration and uncontrolled haemorrhage or to damage of major intrarenal vessels and subsequent infarction. In addition, renal biopsy in man may be quite painful, and there is no reason to assume that this is not the case in animals. Although animals with renal disease may not be ideal candidates for general anaesthesia, correction of fluid and electrolyte imbalances prior to induction and careful anaesthetic technique usually allow the procedure to be completed safely.

In the case of diffuse renal disease, it is usually easiest to

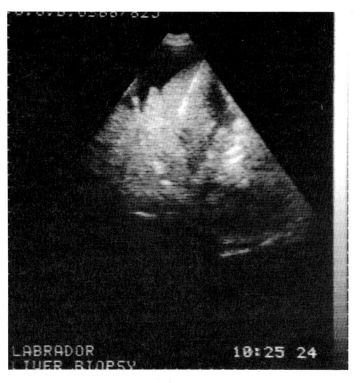

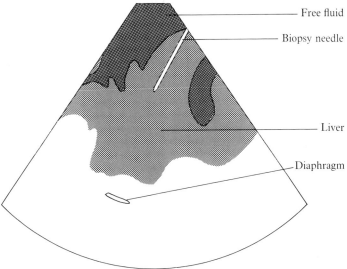

Fig. 10.3 Needle biopsy of the liver under ultrasound guidance.

take the biopsy from the caudal pole of the left kidney as this is the most accessible part. It is important to restrict the biopsy site as far as possible to the renal cortex. There are two main reasons for this: the renal cortex is the important tissue from a diagnostic point of view; and if the arcuate vessels located at the corticomedullary junction are damaged, the risk of serious haemorrhage and/or subsequent infarction is increased. The needle should thus be introduced until it just penetrates the renal cortex. If the needle is introduced too far into the cortex before taking the biopsy, it is likely to pass out through the other side, which increases the risk of haemorrhage and decreases the size of sample obtained. If focal lesions are present, the relevant part of the right or left kidney must be selected, the needle directed to the edge of the lesion and the biopsy taken.

The major contraindications for percutaneous renal biopsy are blood-clotting disorders. It was suggested at one time that acute pyelonephritis was a contraindication for renal biopsy, but experience in human medicine suggests that this is not so. Fluid-filled lesions such as renal cysts, abscesses or hydronephrosis should be sampled by fine needle aspiration and not by core biopsy.

Transient haematuria is a relatively common sequel to renal biopsy. This is usually of little clinical significance. However, formation of blood clots in the renal pelvis has been reported, particularly in cats, and these may be sufficiently large to cause obstruction and hydronephrosis. Intravenous fluid administration before, during or immediately after the biopsy helps prevent clot formation. Restricting the site of the biopsy to the renal cortex should also minimize the risk of this complication. The renal response to injury by needle biopsy has been evaluated in dogs. It has been shown that the ischaemic damage and infarction which occurs secondary to vascular damage may be more extensive than the direct injury of the needle tract. Thus it is important to minimize the number and size of vessels damaged. If a careful biopsy technique is used and the biopsy site is restricted as far as possible to the cortex, the long-term effects are unlikely to be of practical significance. A rare reported complication of renal biopsy is the development of arteriovenous fistulae.

Prostate biopsy

If the prostate gland can be seen clearly ultrasonographically, then it may also be biopsied under ultrasound guidance. The procedure can be performed under sedation and local anaesthesia or under general anaesthesia. The transducer is placed to one side of the prepuce in front of the pubis to image the prostate. A fine needle can then be introduced to aspirate fluid from a cavitary lesion or a biopsy needle can be used to collect a core of solid tissue for histological examination. If a core biopsy is being collected, it is important to avoid damage to the prostatic urethra. It is usually sufficient to direct the needle away from the middle of the gland, but in cases of gross prostatic asymmetry or distortion, it may be useful to place an air- or fluid-filled urethral catheter *in situ* to act as a urethral marker.

Transient haematuria has been reported following prostatic biopsy, but this is rarely of clinical significance.

It is important to become thoroughly familiar with the technique of ultrasound-guided biopsy by practising on cadavers before attempting the procedure on clinical cases. Assuming careful technique, it is a safe and relatively non-invasive method of collecting fluid or tissue samples from internal organs, which may allow a definitive diagnosis to be made. It is also a method which may be performed sequentially to allow monitoring of the progression or resolution of a disease.

Further reading

Finco, D.R. (1974). Prostate gland biopsy. *Veterinary Clinics of North America: Small Animal Practice*, **4**, 367–375.

Hager, D.A., Nyland, T.G. and Fisher, P. (1985). Ultrasound guided biopsy of the canine liver, kidney and prostate. *Veterinary Radiology*, **26**, 82–88.

Hoppe, F.E., Hager, D.A., Poulos, P.W., Ekman, S. and Lindgren, P.G. (1986). A comparison of manual and automatic ultrasound guided biopsy techniques. *Veterinary Radiology*, **27**, 99–101.

Osborne, C.A. (1974). General principles of biopsy. *Veterinary Clinics of North America: Small Animal Practice*, **4**, 213–232.

Osborne, C.A., Hardy, R.M., Stevens, J.B. and Perman, V. (1974). Liver biopsy. *Veterinary Clinics of North America: Small Animal Practice*, **4**, 333–350.

Osborne, C.A., Perman, V. and Stevens, J.B. (1974). Needle biopsy of the spleen. *Veterinary Clinics of North America: Small Animal Practice*, **4**, 311–316.

Papageorges, M., Gavin, P.R., Sande, R.D. and Barbee, D.D. (1988). Ultrasound-guided fine-needle aspiration. *Veterinary Radiology*, **29**, 269–271.

Smith, S. (1985). Ultrasound guided biopsy. *Veterinary Clinics of North America: Small Animal Practice*, **15**, 1249–1262.

Index